a guide to
pilates

Louise Thorley

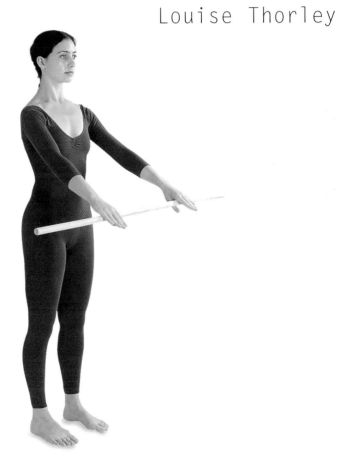

p

This is a Parragon Publishing Book

First published in 2002

Parragon Publishing

Queen Street House

4 Queen Street

Bath BA1 1HE, UK

ISBN: 0-75257-200-8

Printed in China

Designed and created with the Bridgewater Book Company Ltd.

NOTE

Any information given in this book is not intended to be taken as a replacement for medical advice. Any person with a condition requiring medical attention should consult a qualified medical practitioner or therapist before beginning this or any other exercise program.

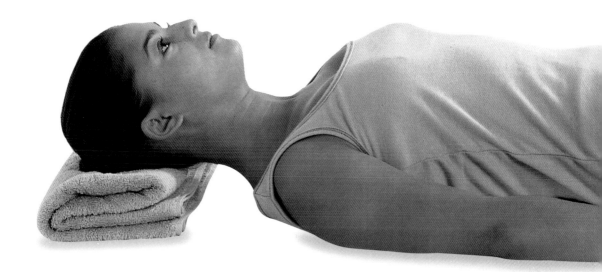

contents

Introduction   4

Part 1: Background

What is Pilates?   6

History and development of Pilates   8

Why do Pilates?   10

How Pilates works   12

Part 2: Preparation

Equipment, environment, and safety   16

Mind and body   20

Learning to breathe correctly   22

Centering the body   26

The importance of good posture   28

Body and movement   32

Part 3: Pilates in Action

Getting into motion   34

Standing exercises   38

Sitting exercises   46

Matwork   50

Glossary   60

Useful addresses and websites   63

Index   64

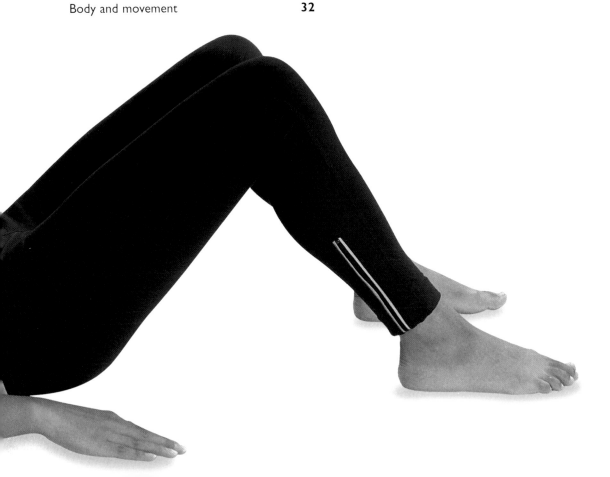

Introduction

Throughout history, people have looked for new and innovative ways to exercise. We can trace yoga to the Indian sub-continent as far back as 4,000 years, and t'ai chi ch'uan, a flowing form of movement, to the China of 2,000 years ago. Developed in the 20th century, Pilates combines ancient wisdom with contemporary knowledge.

The Olympic Games, which started in Greece around the 8th century BCE, attracted athletes from all over the world. Although the games were stopped in 393 CE, their revival in 1896 once again put them in the spotlight. They continue to attract top athletes today and the Games

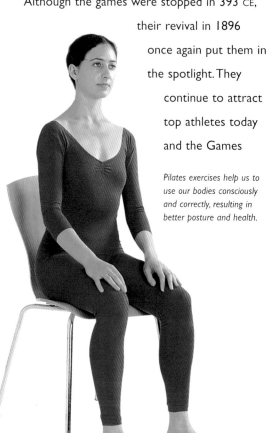

Pilates exercises help us to use our bodies consciously and correctly, resulting in better posture and health.

held every four years are a world event. Like the Games, many ancient forms of exercise are still widely appreciated today, but all over the globe people have continued to find new and fascinating ways to keep their bodies in top condition, from competitive sports such as football, netball and ice hockey, to the new body conditioning systems, including weight-training and aerobics.

The aim of Pilates

The Pilates system of exercise was developed in the 20th century. Practiced regularly, it helps to keep the mind and body working in harmony because it requires a focused mind as well as flowing physical movements. The aim of Pilates is to work different muscles to tone and condition the body, while developing correct breathing, good posture and mental concentration and focus. It improves overall balance and coordination while it streamlines the body and also helps to improve flexibility in all the muscles and joints.

Pilates for everyone

Since it began, this mind-body system of exercise has attracted many rich and famous people from around the world, and it is popular among many Hollywood celebrities. Since the actor Gregory Peck first embraced the teachings of Pilates, many others have followed suit. Today, stars such as tennis player Pat Cash and pop singer Madonna have adopted Pilates as their favored system of exercise. Top models, dancers, and sportspeople have all reaped the benefits of practicing Pilates. Yet the good thing about Pilates is that you do not have to be an athlete to do it. The exercises are gentle and are designed to put as little strain on the body as possible. This means that almost anyone of any age and level of fitness can do it. Whether you are young or elderly, a fitness fanatic or someone who hasn't exercised for years, you can reap the benefits of Pilates. You do not need any equipment either—you can do Pilates in your own home.

*Almost anyone can do Pilates;
the exercises are gentle and put
minimum strain on the body.*

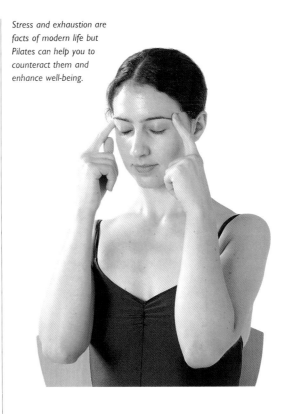

*Stress and exhaustion are
facts of modern life but
Pilates can help you to
counteract them and
enhance well-being.*

Health benefits

Pilates can really improve your health. The carefully designed exercises are very effective for helping you to tone your body and achieve a longer, leaner look and great shape, without creating muscle "bulk." They will help you to reduce stress and beat fatigue, as well as build up your self-confidence and heighten your sense of well-being. You will start to look and feel superb, and move with a new grace that comes from improved coordination and greater muscle flexibility. There is no better time to start reshaping your body—all you need is a little time and the desire to succeed.

What is Pilates?

Pilates is a system of exercise that allows you to take control of your mind and your body. It uses smooth, flowing movements that tone and stretch your body and increase strength and flexibility in your muscles and joints. It also utilizes the power of the mind to help with the exercises and to increase the harmony between body and mind.

Pilates has been referred to as "a yoga-like system that uses machines." Although Joseph Pilates, the founder of this system, did take some of his inspiration from yoga, the exercises are different. If you have a Pilates studio near you which has special apparatus, such as pulleys and springs, these can be helpful but are not essential. Through performing the exercises in this book you will see that the only equipment needed to reach optimum fitness and health is the body itself.

Minimum time, maximum results

Pilates exercises have been designed to work the muscles of the body as efficiently as possible in the minimum time. These low-impact exercises treat the body as a whole and are very effective. There is therefore no need to spend hours each day in the gym: You need to practice only two or three times a week, and can start with 10-minute sessions and build up to longer ones slowly.

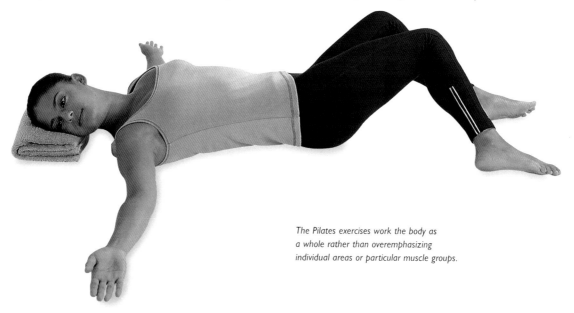

The Pilates exercises work the body as a whole rather than overemphasizing individual areas or particular muscle groups.

Reshaping the body

The capacity of the Pilates exercises to reshape the body has attracted many people from all walks of life over the years. While it is certainly true that this form of exercise can alter your physical appearance, it should be remembered that each person has his or her own individual body shape. It is important to work with what you have already and to recognize that you cannot totally change your shape. The chart below shows how the human body can be classified into three basic shapes, which are known as the ectomorph, the mesomorph and the endomorph.

These shapes help to define how we look, but some people believe that a person's body shape can also be linked to certain personality traits. Some of these are listed below.

Body shapes

Body Type	Ectomorph	Mesomorph	Endomorph
Build	Light and delicate; often tall and thin, with long limbs	Athletic or muscular; large chest, limbs and muscles	Heavy or rounded; may have trouble keeping body weight down
Other Characteristics	Sometimes linked to alertness and an inhibited and intellectual personality	Sometimes associated with an aggressive tendency; mesomorphs are often athletic and can excel at many different sports	Quite often linked to placidity, as well as a relaxed attitude and hedonism

History and development of Pilates

The Pilates system was developed by a German called Joseph H. Pilates. He suffered from rickets and other illnesses as a child and grew up determined to strengthen his weak body. His interest in fitness was fueled during the First World War, when he served as an orderly and became involved in the treatment of patients who were immobile.

During the 1920s, Pilates developed a series of exercises that used various pieces of apparatus to increase efficiency. For example, he devised exercises that patients could perform in bed and he attached springs to their beds in order to increase the efficiency of the exercises. He quickly noticed that patients recovered more quickly when the springs were used. In fact, those springs became the first part of his extensive exercise equipment and he went on to develop many more.

Good balance is an integral part of Pilates, and the system includes standing exercises that can be practiced anywhere, at any time.

After the War

When the First World War came to an end, Pilates moved to America and opened a fitness studio in New York. His techniques soon attracted the interest of famous, wealthy and influential people. He went on to develop and perfect his methods, and continued doing so for the rest of his life. Although he often used pieces of apparatus in his exercises, his original system was based on matwork and was every bit as efficient as his later equipment-based exercises. Pilates' core principles concentrate on rhythmic breathing, a centered posture, flowing, smooth movements and a focused mind.

A simple piece of equipment, such as a broom handle, is used in some exercises to help you to train your body to move correctly.

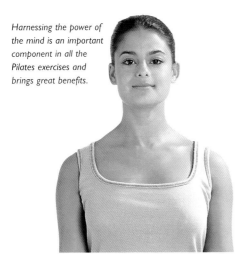

Harnessing the power of the mind is an important component in all the Pilates exercises and brings great benefits.

people to achieve better balance, muscle coordination and graceful movement, as well as increased stamina and flexibility. No wonder it is popular with so many sportspeople today. Many of them have adapted Pilates techniques for their own use and there is no doubt that more and more ingenious ideas, based on Pilates' original principles, continue to flourish.

Pilates today

Originally there were 34 Pilates movements but over the years different practitioners and teachers have brought in their own modifications of these very powerful techniques. As a result, there is no one true system anymore: people have introduced their own ideas and innovations over the decades, so that the whole practice of Pilates has evolved and brought with it other exercises and modifications of earlier ones. However, they still conform to the basic principles behind the original system.

One of the best things about Pilates, however, is its flexibility. Once you know how the system works, you can translate its movements for use into other systems, and many people use it to enhance their work in other disciplines. The exercises can help

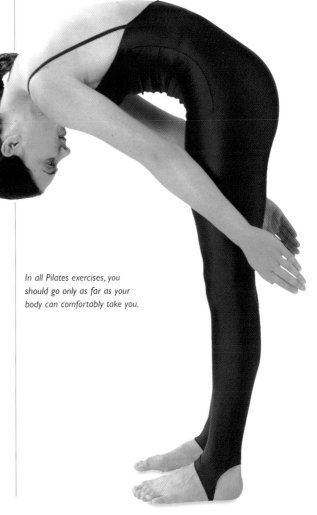

In all Pilates exercises, you should go only as far as your body can comfortably take you.

Why do Pilates?

The Pilates system offers a complete work-out for the body that exercises not just the main muscle groups, but weaker, less-used muscles too. It therefore enables you to achieve a perfectly toned body and realize your true fitness potential. It is also an exercise system that is open to all, because anyone of any age can do Pilates.

Benefits

There are enormous rewards to be gained from doing Pilates regularly. In addition to greater self-confidence and an increased sense of well-being, practicing Pilates can offer the following advantages:

Improved balance: The exercises give you a greater understanding of your body and muscular systems. You will become more aware of the symmetry of your body and how every movement has its own balances and checks.

Less stress: Pilates enables you to relax, and also to work off the chemical effects of stress, such as excess adrenaline in the body.

More efficient digestion: Pilates can help to tone and strengthen the muscles of the stomach. Since it also helps to reduce stress, this will help to ease the digestive process, which shuts down during times of severe stress and tension.

Increased oxygen intake: This helps the body's systems to function efficiently, resulting in clearer thinking, greater energy levels and muscular health.

Better circulation: Pilates helps to improve blood flow, which means more efficient circulation of nutrients and oxygen, and easier removal of toxins.

Improved skin: Improved cardiovascular function means more efficient removal of waste products and a clearer skin.

Enhanced immune system: Pilates exercises the muscles, which helps lymph to circulate around the body. Lymph carries white blood cells, which fight disease.

Sculpted body: The exercises help you achieve a longer, leaner look.

Greater strength and coordination: As you practice, your coordination, strength and balance will increase. You will move with greater ease and grace.

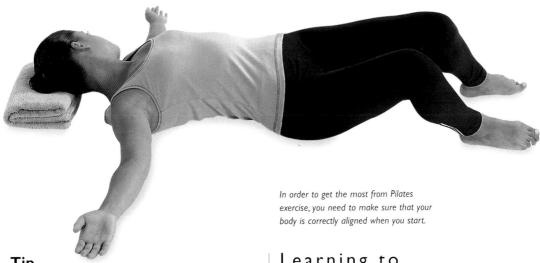

In order to get the most from Pilates exercise, you need to make sure that your body is correctly aligned when you start.

Tip

The best physical fitness programs are those that improve flexibility, build strength and increase stamina. Pilates helps you to build your strength and flexibility, and improves your muscular coordination, but to get the maximum results you should combine your Pilates program with a form of cardiovascular exercise, such as aerobics, in order to build up stamina.

Make sure that your movements are slow and smooth and that your mind is focused when you practice Pilates.

Learning to practice Pilates

This book provides a basic introduction to Pilates, and will be useful to anyone who wants to find out more about Pilates and learn how to do some of the basic exercises. It is particularly suitable for people in reasonable health who have no medical conditions or physical injuries. If you do have a medical condition or injury, however, or you are in any doubt whatsoever about your level of fitness or the suitability of Pilates exercises for you, you should consult your doctor or other qualified medical practitioner before you begin. This book is also not intended to be a substitute for training with a qualified Pilates teacher, and if you decide to explore this system of exercise further, we would strongly recommend that you seek out classes with a suitably qualified instructor in your local area (see page 63).

How Pilates works

Pilates exercises work on the body in a very effective way. Rather than isolating particular muscle groups, they work on the body as a whole, equipping you to perform everyday tasks more efficiently, such as carrying shopping, gardening, and moving furniture. Practicing Pilates will also enable you to become more supple and flexible.

Emotions

Practicing Pilates can contribute to good health on an emotional level as well as a physical one. It can increase your self-confidence and enhance your sense of well-being. It can also reduce your stress levels and help you to be more relaxed.

In a life-threatening situation, or in other circumstances that cause a lot of stress, the stress response, or "fight-or-flight mechanism" as it is known, is activated in your body. As your body gears up to meet the immediate threat, adrenaline is released, the heartbeat, metabolism and breathing become more rapid, and cortisol and other hormones are circulated round the system. Any function that is not essential to immediate survival—including the immune system and digestion—is automatically shut down.

This fight-or-flight response helped our ancestors to run away from predators, preparing the body for physical effort. The physical exertion involved in running away or

Pilates and the body

Pilates is an excellent body-toning and conditioning system of exercise and works on the body on many different levels:

- Emotions
- Nerves
- Tissue
- Muscles
- Bones

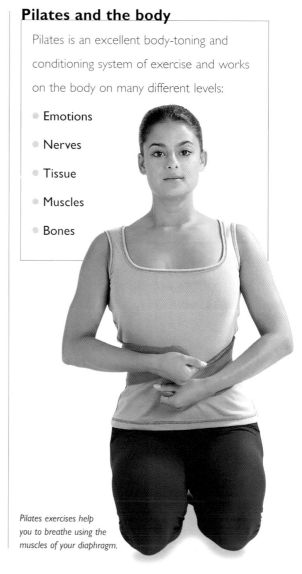

Pilates exercises help you to breathe using the muscles of your diaphragm.

fighting released the stress. Once the immediate danger was over and the effort had passed, the body would return to normal.

Nowadays, we cannot always use physical exertion to counter the stress response. So the stress chemicals stay in the body, draining energy and hampering the digestion and the immune system. Pilates helps to reduce the stress response, enabling our bodies to function normally. Breathing is more relaxed, the heartbeat is slower and steadier, and the metabolic process is more regular. We digest our food more easily, and are less susceptible to colds. As we begin to feel more relaxed, our mood improves and we feel happier.

Tissue

Pilates exercises can help to tone the connective tissue that surrounds, protects and supports vital body parts, including bones, tendons and muscles. Regular practice of Pilates over a period of time can strengthen this tissue, which will enhance coordination of movement and reduce the risk of injury.

Nerves

At the center of the nervous system are the brain and spinal cord, but the nervous system is in fact a vast network of cells that carry information between all the parts of the body in order to control the body's activities. It is

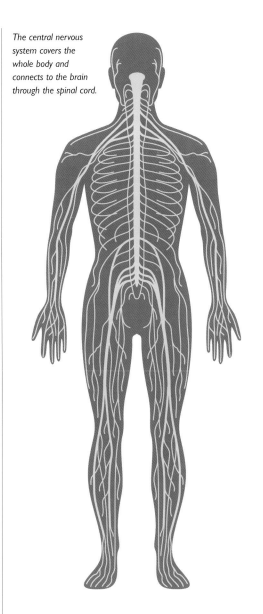

The central nervous system covers the whole body and connects to the brain through the spinal cord.

responsible for movement and coordination. Nerve impulses are sent to and from the brain and tell us how we feel. They also coordinate our movements. Pilates helps us to find a balance between relaxation and tension, and to develop awareness of the nervous system.

Muscles

There are over 650 muscles in the body and they do a huge amount of work. They enable the body to move, they allow us to sit and stand, and they control key body functions. The heart, for example, is a large muscle that pumps blood round the body. The stomach and intestines are also muscles that are responsible for the digestive process. Pilates helps to tone and strengthen these muscles so that they work more effectively.

Isolating one muscle or set of muscles in physical exercise is contrary to the principles of Pilates, however. Pilates concentrates on working the whole body, and in this way prepares it more thoroughly for performing everyday tasks. Muscles often work in pairs or groups anyway, and so concentrating on one muscle will only work to the detriment of another. However, it is a good idea to know where different muscles are situated in the body, so here is a quick reference guide.

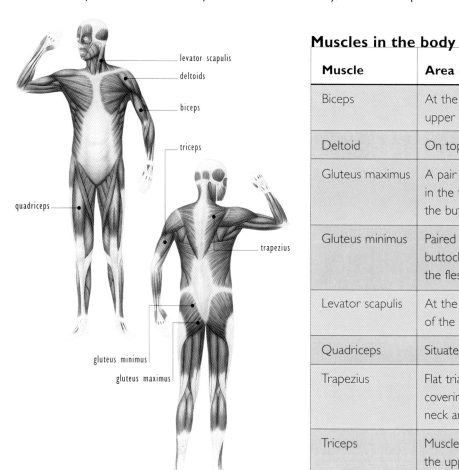

levator scapulis
deltoids
biceps
triceps
quadriceps
trapezius
gluteus minimus
gluteus maximus

Muscles in the body

Muscle	Area of body
Biceps	At the front of the upper arms
Deltoid	On top of the shoulders
Gluteus maximus	A pair of muscles in the fleshy part of the buttocks
Gluteus minimus	Paired muscles in the buttocks just above the fleshy part
Levator scapulis	At the sides and back of the neck
Quadriceps	Situated in the thighs
Trapezius	Flat triangular muscle covering the back of the neck and the shoulder
Triceps	Muscles at the back of the upper arms

Bones

Pilates exercises work to bring the bones of the body back into their natural and correct alignment. With regular practice, this helps to improve posture and coordination of movement. The exercises also increase stability, which in turn enables you to perform physical movements and exercises more efficiently. Regular practice of Pilates can also mobilise joints and keep the whole body working smoothly. This can be especially valuable as you get older, because you will be able to increase your mobility and stay more active well into your later years.

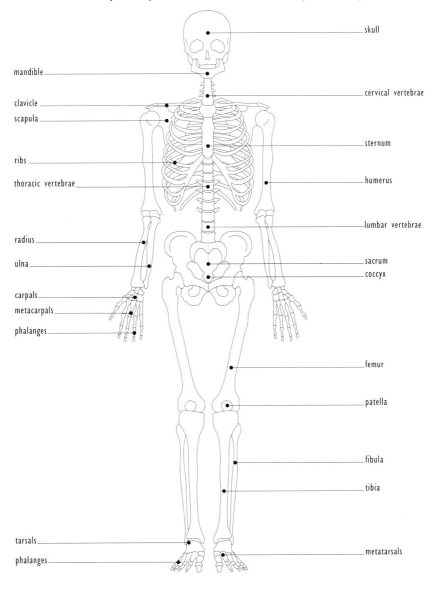

skull

mandible

clavicle

scapula

cervical vertebrae

sternum

ribs

thoracic vertebrae

humerus

radius

ulna

lumbar vertebrae

sacrum

coccyx

carpals

metacarpals

phalanges

femur

patella

fibula

tibia

tarsals

phalanges

metatarsals

Equipment, environment, and safety

Although Joseph Pilates devised many ingenious pieces of equipment to enhance his exercises, and there is no doubt that the apparatus can produce very beneficial results when used in a specific training program, there is no need to purchase any special equipment in order to practice this system of body-conditioning.

Where to practice

If you have a Pilates studio near where you live, this is helpful but not essential. Anyone can practice Pilates in the comfort of their own home. You do not need any special apparatus to do the exercises but you should ensure that your working area is both comfortable and safe. For the floor exercises, a thick carpet or rug that helps to protect your spine is important. As you progress onto the more challenging routines, you may decide that it is worth investing in a thick sports mat, but again this is not essential.

Your working space should be warm enough to keep your muscles relaxed. However, avoid working in very sunny spaces or near sources of artificial heat because your body will become too warm. Ensure that there is a good air supply and that there is no clutter around you or any other obstructions.

A mat protects your spine and helps to keep you warm when exercising on the floor, while a folded towel can be used to aid alignment.

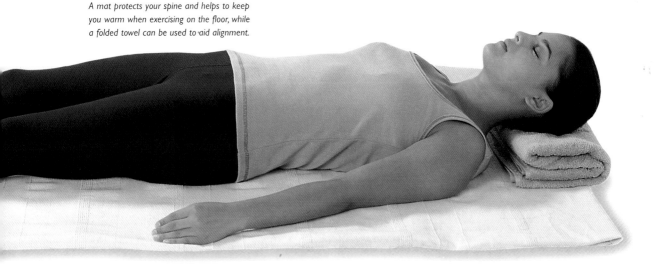

What to wear

Leotards, training shorts and vests are ideal because you can see your muscles as you work them. These are not vital, however, and if you haven't got any working-out gear you can use any comfortable, loose-fitting clothes instead. Avoid any clothing that is tight around the waist. It is preferable to choose something in cotton because it will help to keep you cool. With regard to footwear, you can practice either barefoot or in trainers. Remember to remove your watch and any jewelry before you start.

Timing

You can practice Pilates whenever you feel like it, at any time of day. Some people feel more like exercising first thing in the morning, while others prefer to exercise during the day or in the evening. The choice is yours. However, you should avoid doing Pilates directly after a meal, or if you are tired or feeling unwell.

Exercise sessions can be as short as five minutes or as long as an hour. Some people like to do one daily session of, say, 15–30 minutes, while others prefer to do several shorter sessions in a day. Whatever you decide, the most important thing is to do it regularly, and not to rush. If you only have five or ten minutes to spare, it is better to go for quality rather than quantity, so aim to do a few exercises slowly but well. Never be tempted to rush the movements in order to fit in more repetitions.

If you want to see steady results in a reasonably short time, you should aim to do a 15-minute Pilates session at least four times a week. However, any time you spend doing Pilates will not be wasted. Short sessions during work breaks can be particularly valuable for reducing stress and increasing relaxation.

One of the best things about the Pilates system is its flexibility—you can practice at the time and in the place that suits you best.

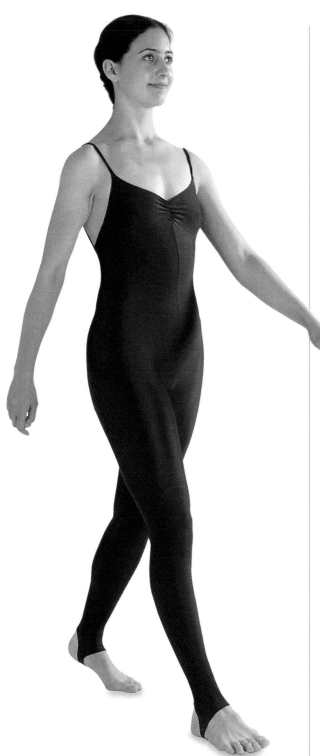

Safety

Whether you are going to do a five-minute session or one hour of Pilates, you must always warm up first to avoid injury. If your muscles are cold they will naturally tense up and this is when injuries are most likely to occur. Walking briskly on the spot or outside for a few minutes will help the body to warm up. There are also warm-up exercises you can do before your workout, and I have given a selection of these later in the book.

If you have an injury or any medical condition, or if you are pregnant or in doubt as to your suitability for exercise, you should seek qualified medical advice before beginning any of the exercises in this book. It is possible to do Pilates while pregnant, but it should only be done after consulting your doctor and under the guidance of a qualified Pilates instructor.

A few of the Pilates exercises can occasionally aggravate some symptoms of menstruation, so if you are in any doubt it is best to avoid it at this time. Also, if you have recently suffered from a minor illness, such as a cold or a throat infection, avoid doing any exercises for at least two weeks after the symptoms have subsided.

It is essential to warm up before a Pilates session to avoid injury; if your muscles are cold and tense, you risk hurting yourself.

Other safety tips

You should always make sure that you drink plenty of water during the day—between 2¾–3½ pints (1.5–2 litres) per day is usually recommended. Never allow yourself to become dehydrated during exercise sessions. When your body is dehydrated, you may suffer from a variety of symptoms including nausea, headache, and exhaustion. An adequate intake of water will help to flush toxins and other waste products from your body, and leave you feeling refreshed and energetic for your exercise session.

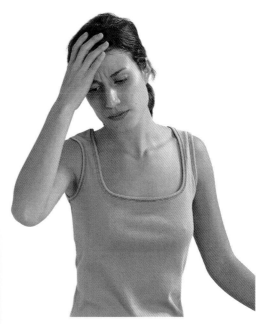

Water helps you to flush toxins from your system; a lack of it can cause headaches, nausea, and tiredness.

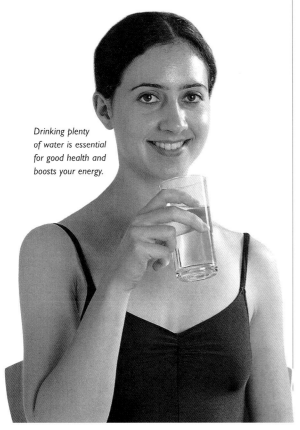

Drinking plenty of water is essential for good health and boosts your energy.

Some of the exercises may feel very gentle on the body at first, but this can be deceptive because their effects may not be felt until the next day. So take it easy, and do not push yourself to the point of discomfort. Never strain, and if you feel any sharp or sudden pain you have overdone it and should ease off at once. There is no hurry and no pressure, so do the exercises in your own time and do not try to do too much too soon.

Finally, after you have finished exercising, try not to stop moving straight away. Keep active for a few minutes, even if it is just tidying up round the home or walking from room to room. This will allow your body time to settle back into its normal rhythm.

Mind and body

One of the key differences between Pilates and many other forms of exercise is that it uses the power of the mind to help with the physical exercises. This mind-body approach has opened up a new realm of possibilities in the world of physical fitness, enabling the body and the mind to work together to create a framework for exercise that is harmonious, balanced, and focused.

Define your goals

Before you begin your new exercise program, it helps to have an idea of just what you hope to achieve. If you want to sculpt your body to make the most of its natural shape, you can do so with Pilates exercises. If you want to be taller, leaner and more supple, you can achieve that too. You can also improve your posture, increase your muscular strength,

Take a little time to focus your mind and think about what you want to achieve from a Pilates program.

and achieve a greater degree of physical flexibility. If you want to be slimmer, Pilates will help you to tone and shape your body, but it won't make you lose weight on its own—you will need to adjust your diet too, and take up some kind of fat-burning exercise to achieve the maximum effects.

So before you start, take some time to decide exactly what you want to achieve from your Pilates workouts, and keep that goal in mind as you practice. Being aware of your goals will help you to achieve them more quickly.

You can create a longer, leaner shape with Pilates, but to achieve consistent weight loss you may have to adjust your diet too.

The power of visualization

The mind has enormous power to bring about changes in the physical body. This is because our bodies do not actually distinguish between things we visualize and reality itself. So if we visualize a stressful situation, for example, and do it so that it feels very real, it will trigger the body's "fight-or-flight" mechanism (see page 12), which will release adrenaline and anti-inflammatory agents into the system, and halt body processes such as digestion. Likewise, if we visualize ourselves experiencing a really joyous occasion, the body will respond accordingly by releasing "happy" chemicals such as endorphins into the system.

You can learn to use the power of visualization to help you while you exercise. For a start, simply visualizing yourself how you want to be will help you to manifest that wish on a physical level. It will also help to keep your motivation up. Practicing visualization can also help you get into the right positions and

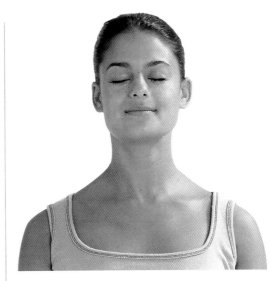

Visualizing a positive reality can help it to come true, so remember to focus your thoughts before, during and after exercise.

to do the exercises correctly. For example, if you imagine that your lower back is anchored to the floor, or that you are pulling in your navel toward your spine, it will help you to work the right muscles and to perform the required movement correctly.

Visualization can therefore be a great ally in any fitness regime—and it costs nothing to incorporate it. You should use it as much as possible to get the quickest and best results.

Imagining that you are pulling your navel toward your spine will help you to isolate and work the correct muscles.

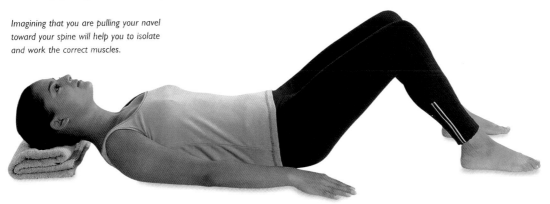

Learning to breathe correctly

Correct breathing is vital to ensure a good flow of oxygen into the lungs: Life-giving oxygen cleanses the bloodstream and energizes the whole body. Although as babies, we naturally breathe correctly, many people develop poor or incorrect breathing habits throughout their lives. The correct technique can be mastered with a little patience.

Benefits of correct breathing

The breath is the very stuff of life and there are many benefits to be gained by learning to breathe correctly. It can:

- Cleanse the bloodstream
- Increase your energy levels
- Carry valuable nutrients to the vital tissues in your body
- Energize your organs and muscles
- Help you to exercise more efficiently
- Aid smooth movement
- Help you to think more clearly
- Enhance muscle control

The importance of rhythmic breathing

When you inhale, you take oxygen into the lungs. The act of breathing also circulates blood around the body. When you exhale, you expel stale air and gases, such as carbon dioxide, from the lungs. If you hold your breath during physical effort, carbon dioxide stays in your lungs. In this way, it accumulates in the body and weakens your muscles. Holding the breath can also increase blood pressure, make you tense and waste energy. This is why it is vital to breathe in a rhythmic and continuous way during exercise.

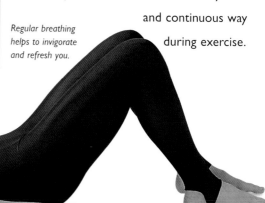

Regular breathing helps to invigorate and refresh you.

Shallow breathing

Many people do not breathe deeply enough. They breathe into the upper chest only and don't get enough life-giving oxygen into the depths of their lungs. It is important to breathe deeply in order to fill the lungs and ensure that enough oxygen is available to energize and purify the body.

Abdominal breathing

Many people have been taught to breathe using the abdomen, which rises and falls with each breath. This ensures a good intake and expulsion of air, but is not suitable for Pilates.

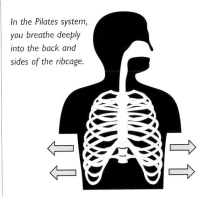

In the Pilates system, you breathe deeply into the back and sides of the ribcage.

Correct breathing— the Pilates way

Joseph Pilates believed that a strong, tight abdomen was a crucial part of his exercise regime, because it gave the whole body the firm stability necessary to perform his workouts. To strengthen the abdomen, however, it is necessary to contract and tighten the abdominal muscles. For this reason, he decided that the abdominal breathing method was not appropriate for practicing his system of exercise. Instead, he decided to use a method called "thoracic breathing," which is also sometimes known as "lateral breathing." This method involves breathing into the back and lower ribs: As the air goes into the lungs, the back and sides of the rib cage expand, then they contract as the air is exhaled. In this way, the abdomen can stay contracted and tight and yet not interfere with the full intake of breath.

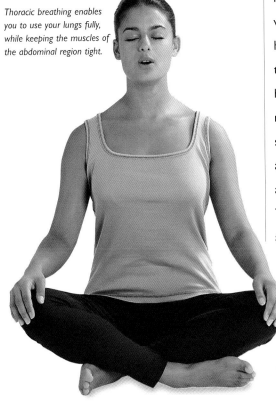

Thoracic breathing enables you to use your lungs fully, while keeping the muscles of the abdominal region tight.

Thoracic breathing

Here is an exercise to help you breathe the Pilates way. It is not difficult to do, but if you have been accustomed to a different method of breathing, it may take a little time for you to get used to it. At first, you will need a long piece of cloth, or a tea towel or scarf, to hold around the bottom of your chest in order to help you perform the movement correctly. When the technique becomes natural to you, you can dispense with the cloth.

1

2

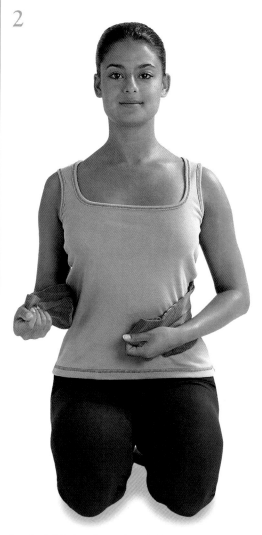

Kneel on the floor. Keep your toes together but let your heels fall naturally apart, then sit back on your heels so that your buttocks are resting on them. Alternatively, sit upright on a chair. Do not let your body rest on the back of the chair—sit up straight.

Place the cloth horizontally around your back and bring the ends round to the front. It should be around your middle, so that you are holding it around the bottom of your chest and ribcage. Keep your shoulders down and let your elbows move out a little from the sides of your body.

Tip

Remember you should exhale on the point of exertion. If you are unsure, just breathe rhythmically—do not hold your breath.

Caution

If you feel unwell or dizzy while you are performing this exercise, stop immediately, loosen the cloth and breathe normally.

3

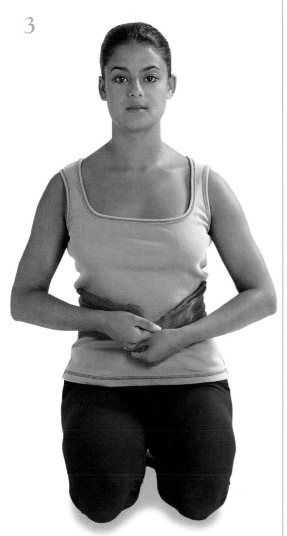

4

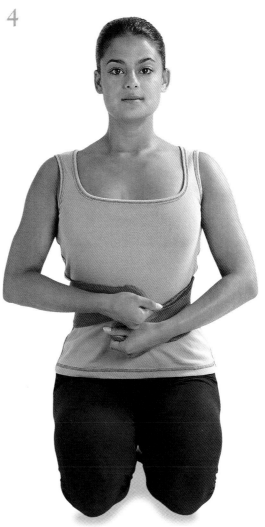

Pull your hands together, pulling the cloth tighter around you as you do so. If necessary, allow your hands to cross over in front of you to ensure that you have a firm hold. However, do not pull the cloth so tightly that it starts to become restrictive or feels uncomfortable.

Take a slow, deep breath, and feel the back and sides of your ribcage push against the cloth. Let the cloth loosen, keeping some resistance. As you exhale, feel your back and the sides of the ribcage contract. Tighten the cloth a little to help empty the lungs. Repeat 8–10 times, then relax.

Centering the body

Joseph Pilates believed that the area from our abdominal muscles to our buttocks is the center of our body. Imagine the area as a band, stretching round the body at the back and the front. He called it the "powerhouse," and devised his exercises so that all energy and effort travel outward from the center of the body.

Pilates was not alone in believing that the abdominal area is the source of bodily strength. In many Oriental disciplines, for example, the source of good health, energy and strength is believed to be located here. Some Chinese systems, such as Traditional Chinese Medicine, *t'ai chi ch'uan,* and *kung fu,* teach that the storehouse of *ch'i* (life energy) is situated at the *t'an tien,* or abdominal area. For physical movements, such as punches,

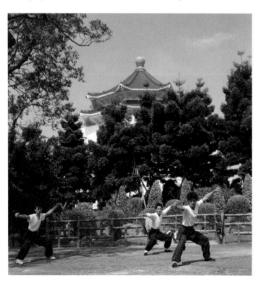

Like Joseph Pilates, practitioners of t'ai chi ch'uan *believe that the abdominal area is the center for movement and energy.*

energy is generated from the abdomen and carried to the arms to give the power needed to make the movement. Likewise, the powerful kicks that are a well-known part of *kung fu* are generated from the abdomen and the hips.

What the powerhouse of your body can do

Think of the powerhouse as the center of your body, from where all your energy and movement flows. When the powerhouse is strengthened, the effects can be very beneficial. The powerhouse can:

- Support the spine

- Bring stability to the center of the body

- Improve balance

- Aid coordination and help you make smooth, flowing movements

- Protect the lower back

- Tone the abdominal muscles and the pelvic floor muscles

- Increase physical strength

Strengthening the powerhouse

To strengthen your own powerhouse, try the following exercise. You can perform it while standing, sitting, or lying down.

Note

Once you have mastered this exercise, you will be able to perform thoracic breathing (see page 23) while keeping a strong center.

1

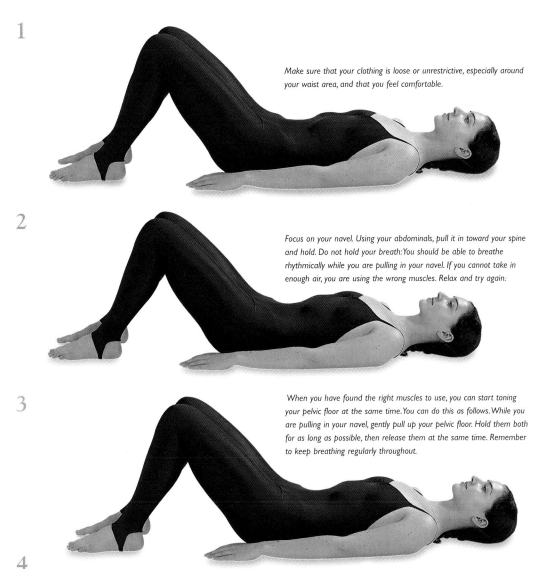

Make sure that your clothing is loose or unrestrictive, especially around your waist area, and that you feel comfortable.

2

Focus on your navel. Using your abdominals, pull it in toward your spine and hold. Do not hold your breath: You should be able to breathe rhythmically while you are pulling in your navel. If you cannot take in enough air, you are using the wrong muscles. Relax and try again.

3

When you have found the right muscles to use, you can start toning your pelvic floor at the same time. You can do this as follows. While you are pulling in your navel, gently pull up your pelvic floor. Hold them both for as long as possible, then release them at the same time. Remember to keep breathing regularly throughout.

4

When you have got used to these movements, you should hold them for as long as you can. You will need to loosen the tension a little, but not completely so that you can keep it up for longer periods, breathing comfortably. As a guide, when you are pulling in your navel, pull it in only one quarter of the way. Similarly, pull up the pelvic floor part of the way so that you can hold the position for increasingly longer periods of time.

The importance of good posture

Good posture is absolutely vital in our daily lives. It can affect our health and the way we function, and it can also have an influence on our bearing, our balance, the way we move and how we appear to others. It can even affect our moods and emotions.

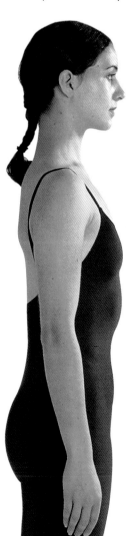

Many people pay little attention to their postural habits until they get back pain or develop some other health problem. Yet with a little perseverance most postural problems can be avoided. Here are just a few of the problems that bad posture can cause:

- Poor circulation
- Neck and back pain
- Muscular strains
- Tension and stress
- Headaches
- Fatigue
- Digestive problems
- Poor muscular movements
- Impaired balance and coordination
- Weakness
- Aching joints

Our postural habits and the body

Over the years, our daily activities and lifestyles cause us to adopt some postures more than others. If we do not know that a particular posture is bad, we will continue to use it until it becomes a habit. Over time, our body shapes "mold" themselves into whatever postures we are adopting, so if we regularly sit slumped or stand incorrectly, our bodies will start to take on that "shape," or compensate for the stress on certain parts of the body by placing exaggerated emphasis on others. The shoulders may become rounded, or the stomach may protrude. By this time, any attempt to sit or stand correctly will be uncomfortable, because the body has begun to mold itself to the incorrect posture.

By the time we reach adulthood, many of us will have started to develop postural problems, especially those relating to the spine. If they continue uncorrected, they can cause a lot of pain in later years.

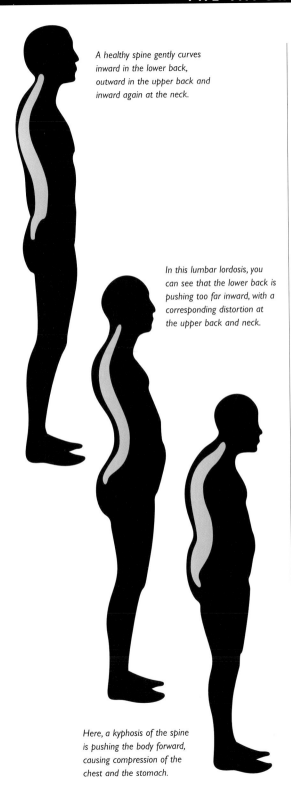

A healthy spine gently curves inward in the lower back, outward in the upper back and inward again at the neck.

In this lumbar lordosis, you can see that the lower back is pushing too far inward, with a corresponding distortion at the upper back and neck.

Here, a kyphosis of the spine is pushing the body forward, causing compression of the chest and the stomach.

Spinal postural problems

One of the main spinal postural problems is lumbar lordosis. Poor posture weakens the abdominals, pulling the stomach forward and creating an unnatural inward curve in the lower back. This causes weakness and pain. The stomach and head drop forward and there is strain on the upper back and neck. The circulation and digestive process are impaired.

In cervical lordosis, the muscles at the back of the neck contract while those at the front expand and the chin protrudes. Over time this condition causes joint inflammation, including arthritis. Another spinal problem, thoracic kyphosis, causes excessive outward curvature of the spine and hunching of the back. This condition can affect the heart, hamper breathing and put strain on the stomach and intestines, resulting in problems with the digestion.

Other spinal problems include thoracic straight spine, caused by contracted muscles; swayback, where the thoracic spine is distorted and muscles are weakened; and visceroptosis, which causes a weak, bloated abdomen and impaired circulation.

Over time, poor posture and bad sitting habits can cause distortions of the spine.

Correcting bad posture

All is not lost, however. Correcting bad posture is perfectly possible, but it takes patience and time for it to become comfortable and natural. Some incorrect postural habits can be sorted out fairly quickly, but of course in some cases the problem will have developed over many years and will need a longer time and more perseverance to put right. The rewards of good posture far outweigh the effort involved, however. Here are just some of the benefits to be gained from correcting your posture:

- Stronger muscles
- Improved functioning of the heart and stomach
- Improved balance and coordination
- Smoother movements
- More efficient circulation, which means nutrients are carried more efficiently to all body systems, resulting in better health, more energy and enhanced appearance
- Strengthened immune system to fight off disease

How to check your posture

It can be quite difficult to know if you are standing or sitting incorrectly. One useful way of checking your posture is to ask someone to take two photographs of you: a side view when you are standing up and a side view of you sitting down. Try not to alter your posture for the camera: just adopt a position that you normally use—one that feels comfortable and natural to you. When you get the photographs, examine them for any "tell-tale" signs of bad postural habits. Here are a few of the most obvious signs you should look out for:

Standing

Rounded upper back

Protruding stomach

Head or chin jutting forward

Slumping

Sitting

Slouching

Rounded shoulders

Compressed chest

Lower back curved outward and compressed abdomen

It is also a good idea to "scan" over your body mentally when you are sitting and standing naturally, perhaps while you are sitting at a desk or standing at the kitchen sink. Work from the top of your head to the bottom of your feet, and try to feel your way through all the muscles and joints. Does any part of your body feel compressed or stretched? Do you feel pain, stiffness, or discomfort anywhere? These symptoms let you know that your posture is incorrect. If you think your posture is incorrect in any way (and it probably will be), you should consult a qualified Pilates instructor or physiotherapist as soon as possible before it has a chance to cause further problems.

A photograph of yourself can give vital clues about your posture.

What Pilates can do

Pilates can help you to find your most efficient and comfortable postures when you are sitting, standing and lying down. Correct postures will also enable you to do the exercises more efficiently and to feel less tired, because there will be less strain on the muscles and body systems. You will be able to breathe more easily, and will feel invigorated and refreshed. The exercises we will be looking at involve standing, sitting, and lying down. Before you start each set of exercises, there will be clear guidelines for you to follow to help you find the right posture.

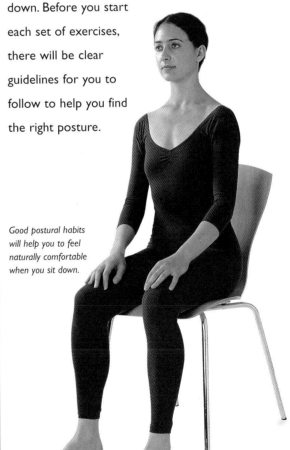

Good postural habits will help you to feel naturally comfortable when you sit down.

Body and movement

Learning to move correctly and at the right pace is an important part of any Pilates physical fitness program. Correct movement and coordination will help you to get the maximum benefit out of the exercises and lessen the risk of injury.

The need to relax

Human beings tend to use short, sharp movements, which appear very jerky when compared with the movements of more graceful mammals, such as cats. This is because humans tend to be tense while they are moving, whereas cats are naturally relaxed.

Too much tension restricts movement and exposes the body to injury. When we are tense, we need to use more energy to get into motion, and expending too much energy over a period of time can lead to fatigue and place an unnecessary strain on the body's systems. We need to be economical with our energy, and not squander it unnecessarily.

So try to cultivate the habit of relaxing when you move. Regularly scan your body both before, during and after movement so that you can keep tension at bay.

Pilates movements

Unlike many forms of exercise, with Pilates you do not pause after each repetition. The movement is continuous, so that one repetition naturally and smoothly flows into the next. The only time that you stop in Pilates is when you come to the end of an exercise.

Slowing the movements down makes the exercises harder to do and more effective. To demonstrate this, try the following exercise.

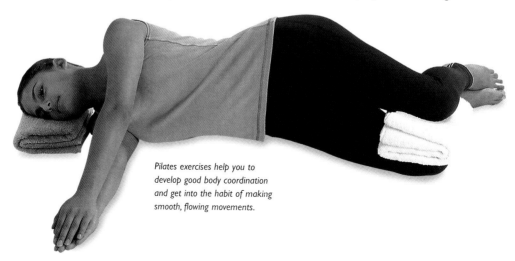

Pilates exercises help you to develop good body coordination and get into the habit of making smooth, flowing movements.

Head lift

Make sure you stay as relaxed as possible while you are performing this exercise. Use a thick carpet or rug to help protect your head and spine. Avoid practicing this exercise if you have a neck problem or neck pain.

If you have done this exercise properly, your neck muscles will feel more tired after step 3 than after step 2, because lifting and lowering your head slowly requires more effort. This is how Pilates exercises work, using slower movements to get the maximum benefit.

1

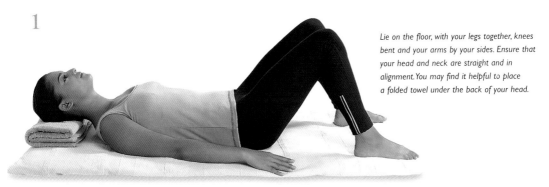

Lie on the floor, with your legs together, knees bent and your arms by your sides. Ensure that your head and neck are straight and in alignment. You may find it helpful to place a folded towel under the back of your head.

2

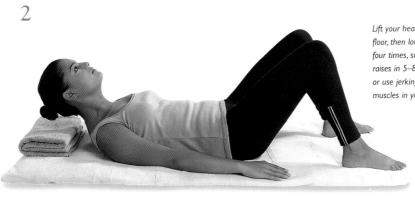

Lift your head 2–2½ inches (5–6 cm) off the floor, then lower it gently back down. Repeat four times, so that you have done about five raises in 5–8 seconds. Do not hold your breath or use jerking movements. Now, how do the muscles in your neck feel? Rest for a minute.

3

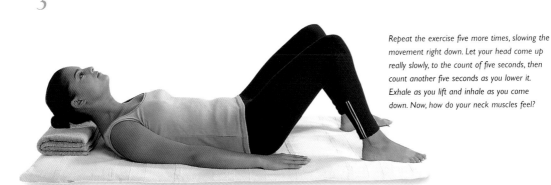

Repeat the exercise five more times, slowing the movement right down. Let your head come up really slowly, to the count of five seconds, then count another five seconds as you lower it. Exhale as you lift and inhale as you come down. Now, how do your neck muscles feel?

Getting into motion

Pilates exercises are many and varied—in fact too many to include here—so the following pages contain a selection of some basic ones to get you started. If you want to explore this system of exercise further, you should find a qualified Pilates teacher who can give you an exercise program suited to your own body and flexibility.

Warming up the body

Before you do any form of physical exercise, you should always warm up your body first. Whether you are going to do a very short ten-minute workout or a longer program, you need to warm up before you begin. This is because when muscles are cold, they are inclined to tense up, which can cause injury.

How to warm up

There are different methods you can use to warm up. For example, you could try walking briskly on the spot or outside for a few minutes to help the body to warm up. Moving around briskly will always get the circulation going and prepare the body for exercise. Never be tempted to warm up the body artificially using a fire or other heat source, however, because the body will get too warm.

You can also do some warm-up exercises to get your circulation going. Here are a few easy ones to get you started.

Arm swings

Do this exercise gently, and use slow, controlled movements.

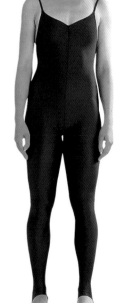

1

Stand up straight, with your feet level and shoulder-width apart and your arms by your sides. Do not lock your knees.

Tip

Remember that you should be drinking plenty of water during the day to avoid dehydrating when you are exercising.

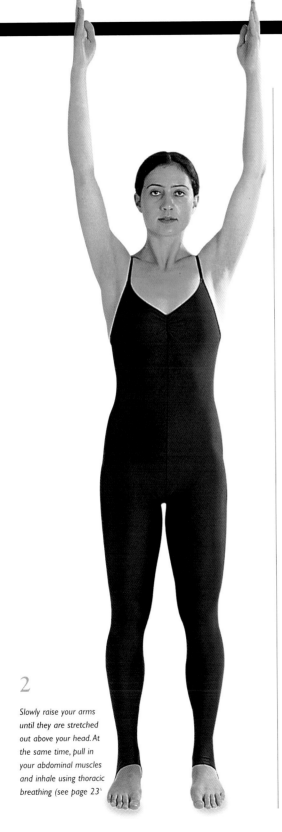

3

Keeping your abdominal muscles tucked in, exhale and swing your arms down past your knees, curling up your body as you do so. Do not let your arms drop: your movement should be slow, controlled, and flowing.

2

Slowly raise your arms until they are stretched out above your head. At the same time, pull in your abdominal muscles and inhale using thoracic breathing (see page 23)

4

Inhale and swing your arms back up above your head, uncurling your body as you do so, until your body and arms are straight. Keep your abdominal muscles pulled in throughout the movement. Do not pause between repetitions: remember that each movement should flow smoothly into the next one. Repeat this exercise 10 times.

Small hoops

This one is good for increasing your heart rate and blood flow. Do not drop your arms as they come down; control the movement.

Large hoops

This exercise is very similar to the previous exercise, but the movements are wider, although still slow and smooth throughout.

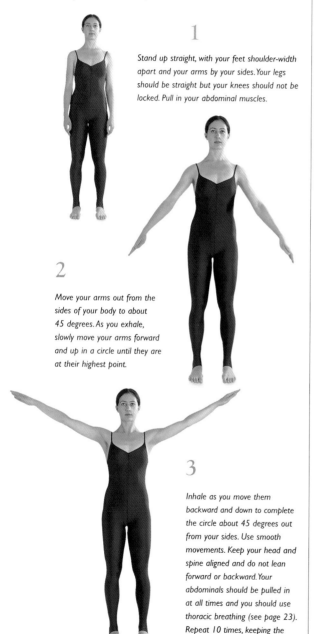

1

Stand up straight, with your feet shoulder-width apart and your arms by your sides. Your legs should be straight but your knees should not be locked. Pull in your abdominal muscles.

2

Move your arms out from the sides of your body to about 45 degrees. As you exhale, slowly move your arms forward and up in a circle until they are at their highest point.

3

Inhale as you move them backward and down to complete the circle about 45 degrees out from your sides. Use smooth movements. Keep your head and spine aligned and do not lean forward or backward. Your abdominals should be pulled in at all times and you should use thoracic breathing (see page 23). Repeat 10 times, keeping the circles the same size.

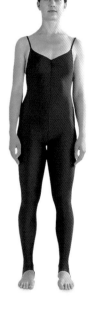

1

Stand up straight, with your feet shoulder-width apart and your arms by your sides. Again, make sure that your legs are straight but that your knees are not locked. Pull in your abdominals throughout the exercise.

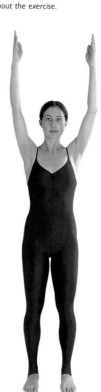

2

Exhale and move your arms forward and up in a wide circle to high above your head. Let your hands touch as you inhale, then move your arms backward and down by your sides to complete the circle. Keep the movements controlled and your head and spine aligned. Do not lean forward or backward. You should use thoracic breathing (see page 23). Repeat this exercise 10 times, keeping the circles the same size.

Progressive hoops

This exercise is similar to the previous hoops exercises, but the movements are in the opposite direction and start off small and get progressively wider. Once again, keep your movements slow and smooth.

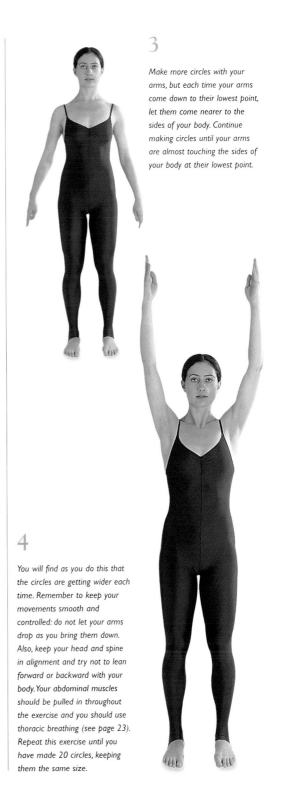

3

Make more circles with your arms, but each time your arms come down to their lowest point, let them come nearer to the sides of your body. Continue making circles until your arms are almost touching the sides of your body at their lowest point.

1

Stand up straight, with feet shoulder-width apart and your arms by your sides. Keep your legs straight but do not lock your knees. Pull in your abdominal muscles throughout the exercise.

4

You will find as you do this that the circles are getting wider each time. Remember to keep your movements smooth and controlled: do not let your arms drop as you bring them down. Also, keep your head and spine in alignment and try not to lean forward or backward with your body. Your abdominal muscles should be pulled in throughout the exercise and you should use thoracic breathing (see page 23). Repeat this exercise until you have made 20 circles, keeping them the same size.

2

Move your arms out from the sides of your body to about 45 degrees. As you exhale, slowly move your arms backward and up in a circle until they are at their highest point, then inhale as you move them forward and down to complete the circle about 45 degrees out from the sides of your body. Keep your head and spine aligned and do not lean forward or backward. Use thoracic breathing (see page 23).

Standing exercises

The following pages focus on exercises you can do while you are standing. In order to do them properly, however, you need to learn how to stand correctly. A good standing posture will help you to perform the exercises more efficiently and improve how your body looks, too. You can appear taller and leaner just by making a few small adjustments to the way you stand.

Getting into good habits

The most effective and quickest way of making good posture become natural to you is to practice it whenever you can. Whenever you are standing or walking, you can practice adopting the right position until it becomes second nature to you.

So wherever you are, whether you are cleaning the home, walking to or from work or around the shops, or even waiting for a bus or train, keep practicing. If you keep forgetting to do it at first, try putting reminders around your home or place of work to help you remember. You could put a sticker next to the bathroom mirror or near the kitchen sink or refrigerator, or you could stick a note on the main door of your home at eye level to remind you to stand correctly whenever you leave your home.

Standing correctly the Pilates way

Finding your correct standing position is a relatively simple procedure, but it may take a little time and practice to sort out any bad postural habits that may have crept in.

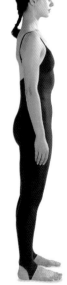

1

Stand up straight, feet shoulder-width apart. Your weight should be evenly distributed over your feet: do not rock onto your toes, backward onto your heels or onto the sides of your feet.

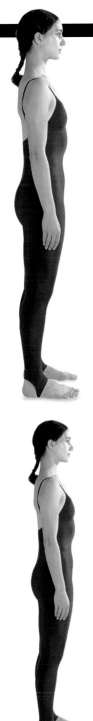

2

Make sure that your legs are straight, and ensure your knees are not locked. Consciously relax the muscles in your lower legs and your thighs.

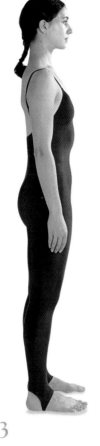

3

Make sure that your powerhouse is strong; pull in your navel and pull up your pelvic floor to about 25 per cent of the tension (see page 27). Keep it at this level for all the exercises in this section.

4

Let the base of your spine fall toward the floor, without moving your pelvis forward. Keep doing the thoracic breathing (see page 23).

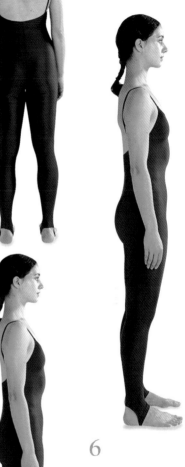

5

Contract and relax your upper back muscles to release tension. Let your shoulders and arms hang naturally.

6

Let your head and neck rest naturally in a central position. You might like to move your head around a little to find this point.

7

Shift your focus to the backs of your ears. Imagine magnets there, pulling upward. Keep doing the thoracic breathing (see page 23) and hold the position for as long as possible.

Arm lifts

This exercise helps you to improve your standing posture by encouraging you to find the right position for your shoulder blades. It also works the muscles in the upper arms.

It may seem a very slow and gentle exercise at first, but as with all Pilates exercises, it is very effective. Keep the movements smooth and controlled.

Caution

Avoid this exercise if you have weak or injured shoulders. If you are in doubt, seek professional medical advice first.

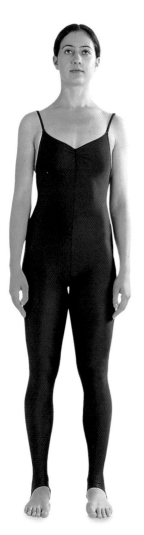

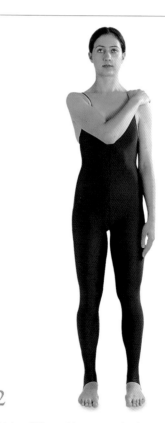

1

Stand tall, feet shoulder-width apart. Make sure that your weight is evenly distributed over your feet, and that your knees are not locked. Pull in your navel toward your spine and pull up on your pelvic floor, holding at 25 per cent tension. Let the base of your spine fall toward the floor, without moving your pelvis forward. Your neck and spine should be aligned, and your hands resting on the outsides of your thighs.

2

Exhale and lift your right arm upward and across your middle until your right palm is resting on the top of your left shoulder. Your left palm at this point should still be resting on the outside of your left thigh. Make sure that you keep breathing in and out rhythmically using the thoracic breathing technique (see page 23) and are maintaining a strong power house, through navel and pelvic floor tension (see page 27).

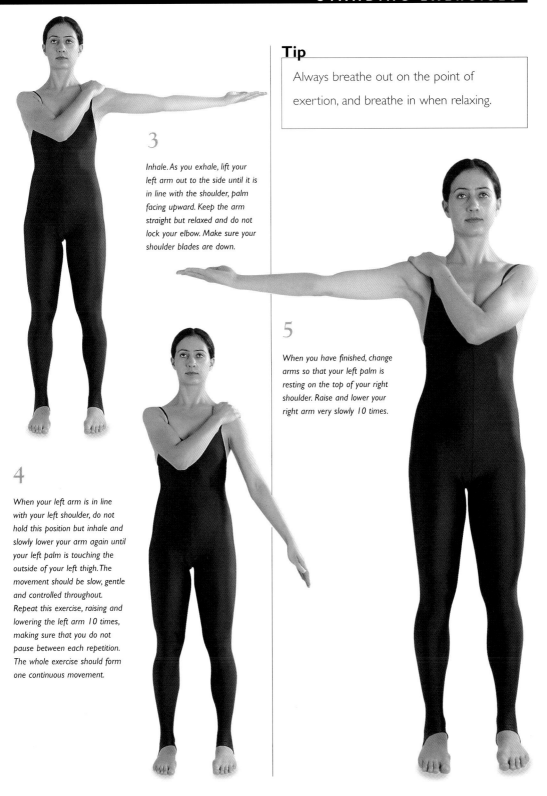

Tip

Always breathe out on the point of exertion, and breathe in when relaxing.

3

Inhale. As you exhale, lift your left arm out to the side until it is in line with the shoulder, palm facing upward. Keep the arm straight but relaxed and do not lock your elbow. Make sure your shoulder blades are down.

5

When you have finished, change arms so that your left palm is resting on the top of your right shoulder. Raise and lower your right arm very slowly 10 times.

4

When your left arm is in line with your left shoulder, do not hold this position but inhale and slowly lower your arm again until your left palm is touching the outside of your left thigh. The movement should be slow, gentle and controlled throughout. Repeat this exercise, raising and lowering the left arm 10 times, making sure that you do not pause between each repetition. The whole exercise should form one continuous movement.

Knee bends and arm lifts

This exercise is relaxing yet invigorating because it helps to get the circulation going. It also helps you to improve your balance and overall stability, while at the same time building on your physical coordination.

Caution

Do not do this exercise if you have weak or injured knees or shoulders. If you are in doubt about its suitability for you, seek professional medical advice first.

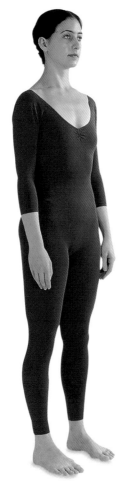

1

Stand up straight, feet shoulder-width apart. Your weight should be evenly distributed over your feet. Keep the legs straight but do not lock your knees. Pull in your navel toward your spine and pull up your pelvic floor muscles, to about 25 per cent tension; let the base of your spine fall toward the floor, without moving the pelvis forward. Keep your neck and spine aligned. Rest your hands on the outsides of your thighs.

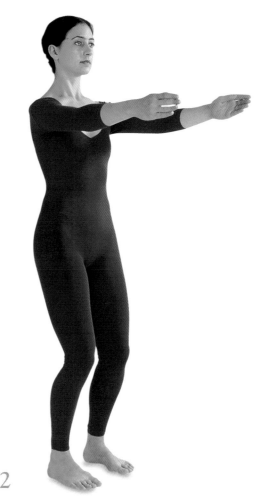

2

Inhale, then as you exhale very slowly lift your arms in front of you to shoulder height. Your palms should be facing each other. Keep your arms straight out in front but do not lock your elbows. At the same time, bend your knees slowly to an angle of about 45 degrees. Keep your weight evenly distributed on your feet: do not rock forward or backward. Don't forget to use the thoracic breathing technique (see page 23).

Tip

Remember to keep pulling in your navel toward your spine throughout this exercise. It will help to protect your back and keep your posture correct and strong.

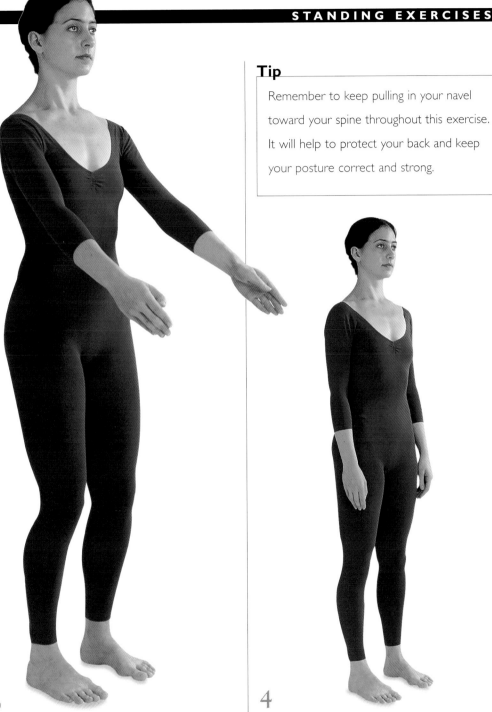

3

When your arms are straight out in front in line with your shoulders, inhale and slowly lower your arms again until your palms are touching the outsides of your thighs. At the same time, straighten your legs until you are standing upright, but do not lock your knees. The movement should be slow, gentle, and controlled throughout.

4

Repeat this exercise, raising and lowering the arms and bending and straightening the knees 10 times, making sure that you do not pause between each repetition. The whole exercise should form one continuous movement throughout. Then, pause and relax for a minute or so.

Chest stretch

The chest stretch helps to develop stability
and good posture while enhancing smooth
movement and coordination. It also gently
stretches and tones the chest, shoulders and
upper arms. You will need a rope or a long
piece of cloth such as a scarf. Alternatively, you
could use a broom handle or other lightweight
pole. Maintain rhythmic breathing throughout,
using the thoracic method (see page 23).

Caution

Avoid this exercise if you have weak or
injured shoulders or neck muscles. If you
are in doubt about its suitability, seek
professional medical advice first.

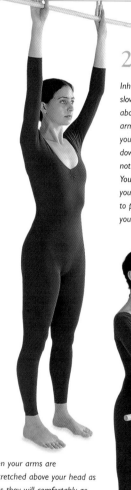

2

*Inhale, then as you exhale very
slowly, lift the pole until it is
above your head. Keep your
arms straight but do not lock
your elbows. Keep your shoulders
down but do not tense them. Do
not let your back arch as you lift.
You should also keep pulling in
your pelvic muscles: this will help
to protect your lower back as
you lift your arms upward.*

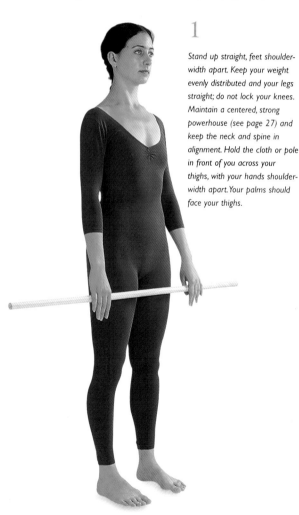

1

*Stand up straight, feet shoulder-
width apart. Keep your weight
evenly distributed and your legs
straight; do not lock your knees.
Maintain a centered, strong
powerhouse (see page 27) and
keep the neck and spine in
alignment. Hold the cloth or pole
in front of you across your
thighs, with your hands shoulder-
width apart. Your palms should
face your thighs.*

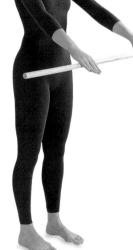

3

*When your arms are
outstretched above your head as
far as they will comfortably go,
inhale and slowly bring them
back down until they are
touching your thighs again. Do
not let your arms drop: keep the
movement slow, gentle, and
controlled. Repeat this exercise
10 times, without pausing
between each repetition.*

Spinal release

This exercise is very effective for releasing tension, improving circulation and increasing flexibility in the spine. You should try to repeat it at the end of your workout too because it is very relaxing and will help you to shake off any remaining tension in your body.

1

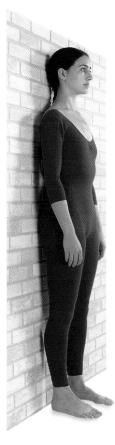

Stand up straight, with your back against a wall and your feet shoulder-width apart. Your weight should be evenly distributed over your feet. Keep your legs straight, but do not lock your knees. Pull your navel in toward your spine, then pull up your pelvic floor muscles and hold at 25 per cent tension. Allow the base of your spine to fall toward the floor, without moving the pelvis forward. Your neck and spine should be aligned. If you can, keep your shoulders in contact with the wall, or get them as near to it as you can without straining. Your heels should be near to the wall but not touching it. Your body should stand straight—if your heels are too far away or too near, your body will curve. Let your arms hang down, hands resting on the outsides of your thighs. Use the thoracic breathing technique (see page 23).

Caution

Do not attempt this if you have high or low blood pressure. If you feel pain, tingling or dizziness, stop and seek medical advice.

2

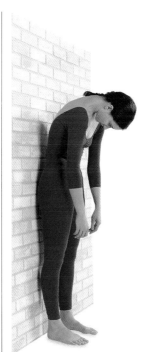

Exhale, and very slowly let your chin drop down toward your collarbone. The movement should be controlled and gentle, so do not let your chin fall heavily. Continue the slow movement downward by gradually letting your shoulders come off the wall, then letting your body roll down slowly, bending down from your shoulders and then from your waist. Roll down as far as you can, keeping your buttocks in contact with the wall. Let your head and arms hang down.

3

When you have bent down as far as you can comfortably go, inhale and then gradually straighten up, unrolling your body bit by bit. The whole movement should be slow and smooth. When you have returned to your starting position, take a couple of moments to check your posture (see step 1). Repeat six times.

Sitting exercises

In this section we will be looking at several different exercises you can do while you are sitting down. Once again, good posture is vital here. Practiced correctly, these exercises will help all your body systems to function more efficiently, which in turn will improve your health and lead to a greater sense of well-being.

Learning how to sit correctly

You can practice correct posture whenever you are sitting down—such as when you are traveling or working. If your job involves hours of sitting in front of a computer or at a checkout, use the time to develop good habits. You can also practice when sitting watching the TV, eating in a restaurant or at the theater. Eventually sitting correctly will become natural.

Sitting correctly the Pilates way

Adopting a good sitting posture is not difficult, but if you have developed bad habits, such as slumping while sitting, it may take practice. For this exercise you will need a chair.

Tip

Your lower back should not arch too much, either forward or backward. Sit sideways in front of a mirror so you can check.

1

Sit upright with your lower back supported against the back of the chair. Do not lean your upper back into the chair and try not to slump or lean forward; you should sit erect but not bolt upright or you will not be able to sit comfortably for long periods of time.

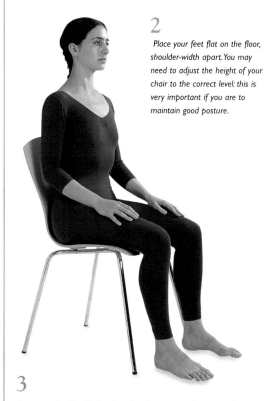

2

Place your feet flat on the floor, shoulder-width apart. You may need to adjust the height of your chair to the correct level: this is very important if you are to maintain good posture.

3

Keep your shoulder blades down, but do not strain. Put your palms on your thighs and do not lean back into the chair. Your head, neck, and spine should be aligned and your head central. Keep your powerhouse strong by pulling in your navel toward your spine and pulling up your pelvic floor muscles, holding at 25 per cent tension.

Side stretches

These stretches are good for getting the lower back moving and for toning the waist. You need a chair with a straight back.

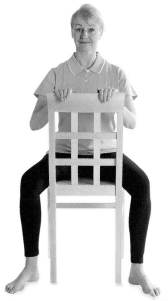

1

Sit facing the chair's back, legs straddling the chair. Make sure that you are sitting erect: your body should not be leaning. Put your palms on the top of the chair's back, keep your arms relaxed, and ensure that your feet are flat on the floor. Pull in your navel toward your spine and pull up your pelvic floor muscles, holding them at about 25 per cent of the tension throughout this exercise. Breathe rhythmically, using thoracic breathing (see page 23).

2

Exhale, stretch your left arm out to the left and raise it to shoulder height, palm upward. Keep raising your arm until it is over your head, palm facing inward. At the same time, move your right shoulder downward so you are leaning to the right.

3

Feel the stretch down your left side. When you have leant over as far as is comfortable, breathe in and straighten up slowly, resting your palm on the chair back again. Repeat on the other side. Then repeat this exercise 10 times.

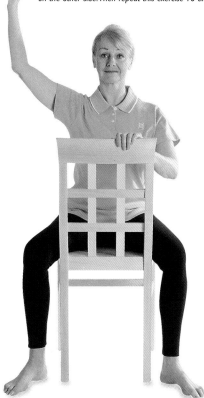

Tip

Remember not to pause between repetitions but to keep your movements slow, continuous, and as smooth as possible.

Spinal twists

This gentle exercise helps to increase the flexibility of your spine, especially in the lower back area. You will need a stool or chair without arms to practice this exercise.

1

Sit erect on the stool or chair. Put your feet flat on the floor, shoulder-width apart, and place your palms on your thighs. Pull in your navel toward your spine and pull up your pelvic floor muscles. Hold at 25 per cent of the tension throughout this exercise. Breathe rhythmically, using thoracic breathing (see page 23).

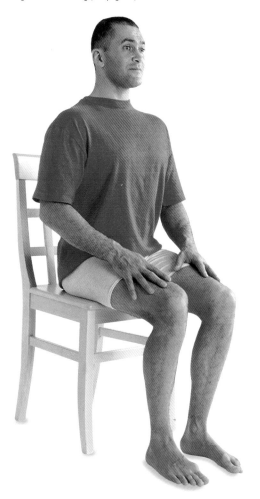

Caution

Do not do this exercise if you have a weak or injured lower back or neck.

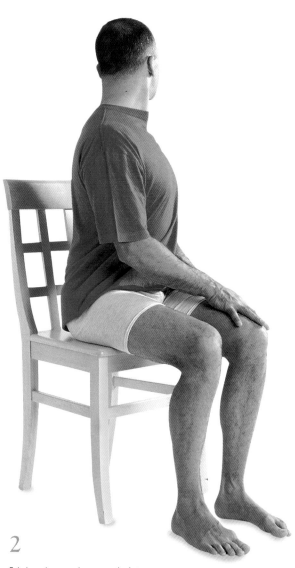

2

Exhale and, as you do so, very slowly turn your head to the left so that you are looking over your left shoulder. As your head turns, let your spine follow the turn to give more of a twist. Move your right hand and place your right palm on your left thigh next to your left hand.

3

When you have twisted round as far as is comfortable, inhale and slowly start to unwind, starting with your head and then letting your spine follow. At the same time, move your right hand back to its original position. You should now be facing the front again.

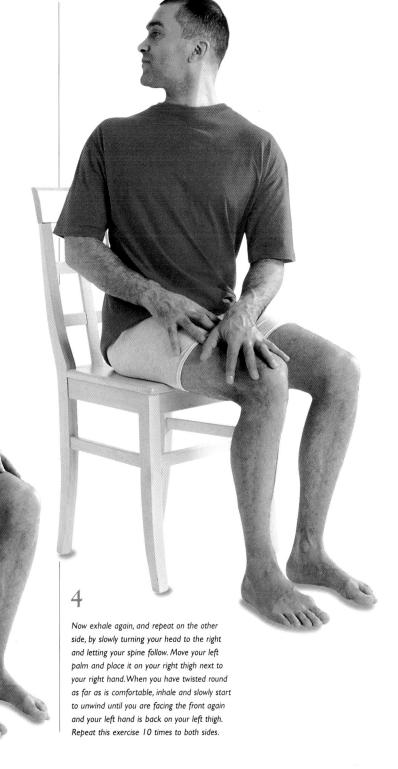

4

Now exhale again, and repeat on the other side, by slowly turning your head to the right and letting your spine follow. Move your left palm and place it on your right thigh next to your right hand. When you have twisted round as far as is comfortable, inhale and slowly start to unwind until you are facing the front again and your left hand is back on your left thigh. Repeat this exercise 10 times to both sides.

Matwork

Most workouts in the Pilates system focus on matwork, or floor exercises. In this section we will look at some of the exercises you can do on the floor. There are many others, so if you would like to explore Pilates further, we would recommend that you seek out a qualified Pilates instructor or studio near to you (some useful addresses and websites are given on page 63). When you have finished these exercises, try doing the Spinal twists again (see pages 48–49), to release any remaining tension.

Equipment

You do not need any special equipment for these exercises, but you will need to practice them on a thick carpet or rug to help protect your spine. As you progress onto a more challenging program, you may decide to buy a thick sports mat, but this is not essential. For these exercises, you will also need a couple of small cushions or pillows, or two small towels that you can fold easily.

Correct posture

Adopting and maintaining the correct posture is just as important for matwork as it is for the standing and sitting exercises. It will enable all your body systems to function at optimum efficiency, so that you can get the most benefit out of your exercise program. For all the floor exercises, you need to make sure your spine and pelvis are in "neutral"; the exercise on page 51 shows you how to do this.

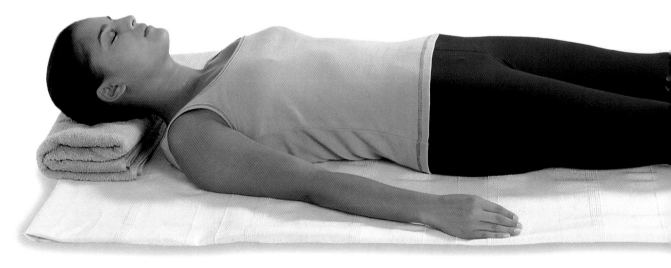

Neutral spine and pelvis

This method will help you to find the most relaxing position for your spine and pelvis while you are working on the floor. You will need a small pillow or cushion, or a small folded towel, to place under your head.

Caution

If you feel any discomfort or pain in your lower back while you are doing this exercise, stop immediately and seek advice from your doctor or another qualified medical practitioner as soon as possible.

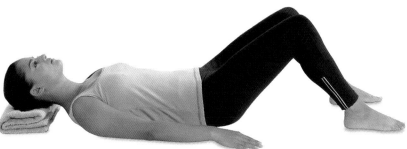

1

Lie on your back on the floor, your head on the pillow or towel. Bend your knees and place your feet on the floor, 10 inches (25 cm) apart. Your palms should be flat and your arms by your sides.

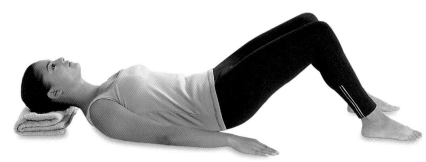

2

Pull in your navel and pull up your pelvic floor, then hold them at 25 per cent of the tension. Breathe rhythmically, using the thoracic breathing method (see page 23). Gently push your lower back toward the floor as far as possible without discomfort. Then relax and let it rise to a comfortable position.

3

Now, arch your lower back by pushing it upward. Do not move your buttocks or upper back from the floor. When you have arched your lower back as far as it will comfortably go, let it sink back gently toward the floor. The neutral position for the spine and pelvis is between these points, neither pushed too low nor arched too high. A slight curve upward is natural: you should be able to slide your hand between your lower back and the floor. Keep your abdominal muscles pulled in. You should maintain your neutral position for your spine and pelvis throughout the floor exercises.

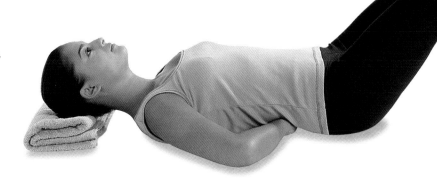

Lumbar twists

These lumbar twists are excellent for improving spinal mobility while keeping your powerhouse strong and centered. You will need a small pillow or folded towel to place under your head for this exercise.

Caution

Do not allow your back to arch excessively, and remember to keep your abdominal muscles pulled in toward your spine.

1

Lie on your back and place your head on the pillow or towel. Bend your knees and put your feet flat on the floor, 10 inches (25 cm) apart. Stretch your arms out to the sides at right-angles to your body, palms facing upward. Do not lock your elbows.

2

Pull in your navel toward your spine and pull up your pelvic floor. Hold them in that position, then release them slightly and hold them at about 25 per cent of the tension. Remember to breathe rhythmically, using the thoracic breathing method (see page 23). You should also have your spine and pelvis in the neutral position (see page 51).

3

Exhale, and slowly turn your head to the right until your right cheek is flat on the pillow or towel. At the same time, very slowly move your knees to the left and let them descend gently toward the floor. If they cannot reach the floor, do not worry; just let them descend as far as they will comfortably go.

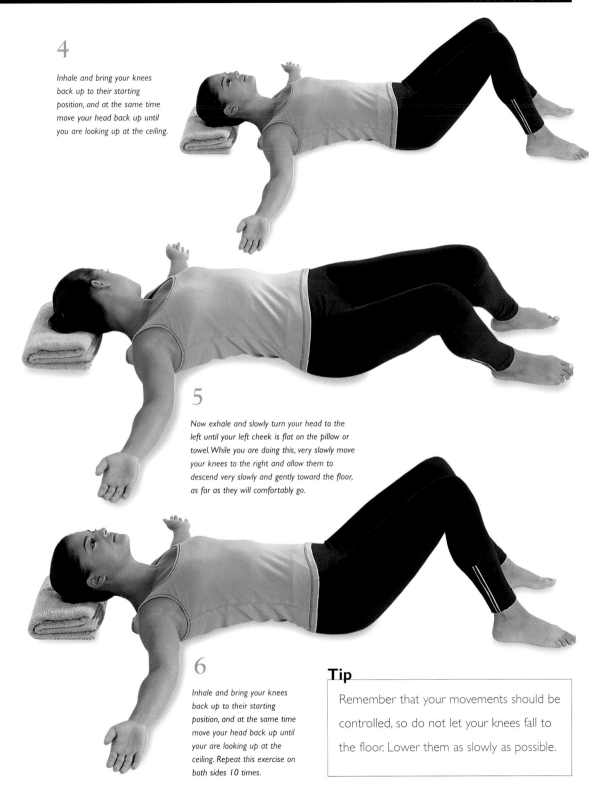

4

Inhale and bring your knees back up to their starting position, and at the same time move your head back up until you are looking up at the ceiling.

5

Now exhale and slowly turn your head to the left until your left cheek is flat on the pillow or towel. While you are doing this, very slowly move your knees to the right and allow them to descend very slowly and gently toward the floor, as far as they will comfortably go.

6

Inhale and bring your knees back up to their starting position, and at the same time move your head back up until your are looking up at the ceiling. Repeat this exercise on both sides 10 times.

Tip

Remember that your movements should be controlled, so do not let your knees fall to the floor. Lower them as slowly as possible.

Chest stretches

This exercise helps you to stretch out your chest and neck muscles, and tones the upper back and spine. You will need two small pillows, cushions, or folded towels.

Caution

Avoid this exercise if you have a weak neck or back or have any injuries in these areas.

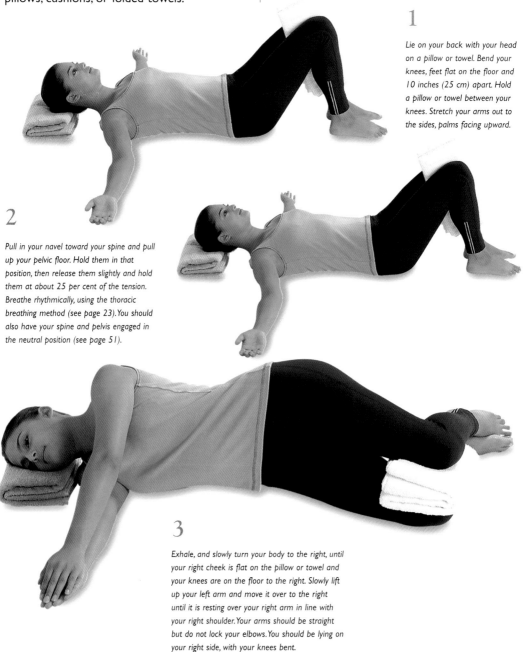

1

Lie on your back with your head on a pillow or towel. Bend your knees, feet flat on the floor and 10 inches (25 cm) apart. Hold a pillow or towel between your knees. Stretch your arms out to the sides, palms facing upward.

2

Pull in your navel toward your spine and pull up your pelvic floor. Hold them in that position, then release them slightly and hold them at about 25 per cent of the tension. Breathe rhythmically, using the thoracic breathing method (see page 23). You should also have your spine and pelvis engaged in the neutral position (see page 51).

3

Exhale, and slowly turn your body to the right, until your right cheek is flat on the pillow or towel and your knees are on the floor to the right. Slowly lift up your left arm and move it over to the right until it is resting over your right arm in line with your right shoulder. Your arms should be straight but do not lock your elbows. You should be lying on your right side, with your knees bent.

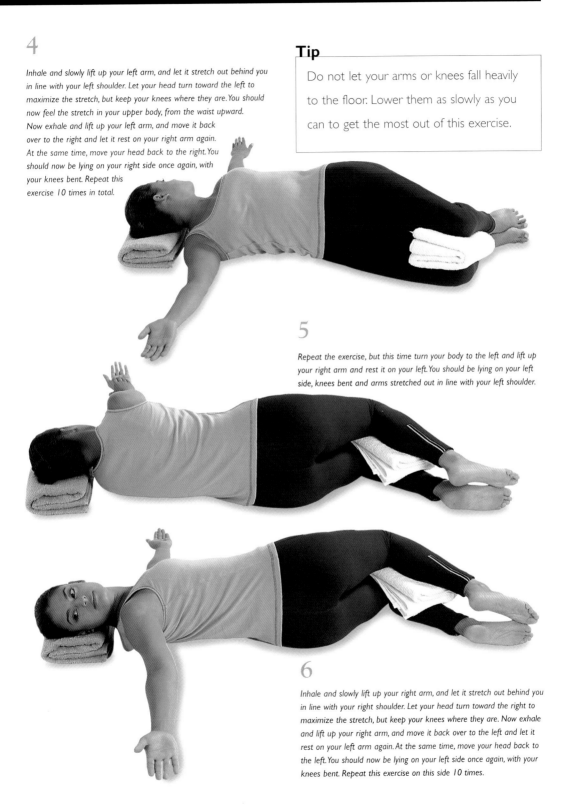

4

Inhale and slowly lift up your left arm, and let it stretch out behind you in line with your left shoulder. Let your head turn toward the left to maximize the stretch, but keep your knees where they are. You should now feel the stretch in your upper body, from the waist upward. Now exhale and lift up your left arm, and move it back over to the right and let it rest on your right arm again. At the same time, move your head back to the right. You should now be lying on your right side once again, with your knees bent. Repeat this exercise 10 times in total.

Tip

Do not let your arms or knees fall heavily to the floor. Lower them as slowly as you can to get the most out of this exercise.

5

Repeat the exercise, but this time turn your body to the left and lift up your right arm and rest it on your left. You should be lying on your left side, knees bent and arms stretched out in line with your left shoulder.

6

Inhale and slowly lift up your right arm, and let it stretch out behind you in line with your right shoulder. Let your head turn toward the right to maximize the stretch, but keep your knees where they are. Now exhale and lift up your right arm, and move it back over to the left and let it rest on your left arm again. At the same time, move your head back to the left. You should now be lying on your left side once again, with your knees bent. Repeat this exercise on this side 10 times.

Backward swimming

This exercise helps to improve muscular coordination and provides a healthy stretch for the legs, arms and stomach. You will need a small pillow, cushion, or folded towel.

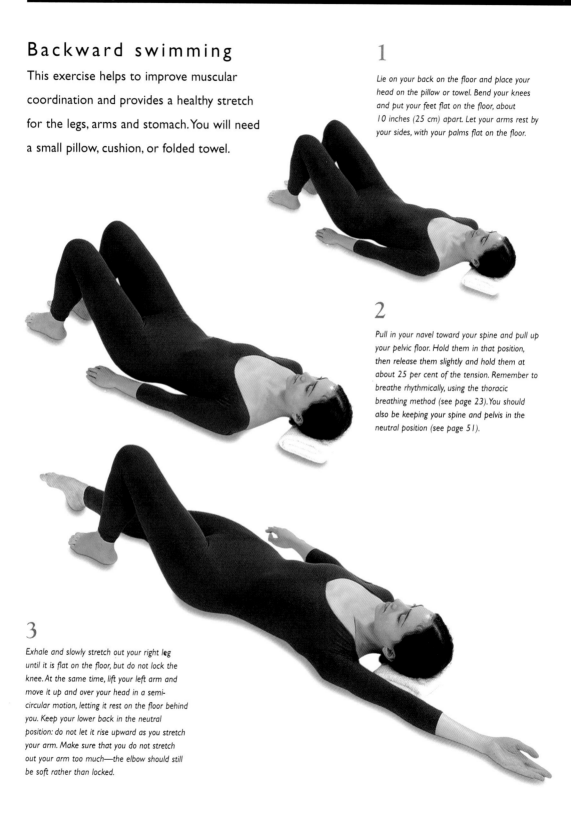

1

Lie on your back on the floor and place your head on the pillow or towel. Bend your knees and put your feet flat on the floor, about 10 inches (25 cm) apart. Let your arms rest by your sides, with your palms flat on the floor.

2

Pull in your navel toward your spine and pull up your pelvic floor. Hold them in that position, then release them slightly and hold them at about 25 per cent of the tension. Remember to breathe rhythmically, using the thoracic breathing method (see page 23). You should also be keeping your spine and pelvis in the neutral position (see page 51).

3

Exhale and slowly stretch out your right leg until it is flat on the floor, but do not lock the knee. At the same time, lift your left arm and move it up and over your head in a semi-circular motion, letting it rest on the floor behind you. Keep your lower back in the neutral position: do not let it rise upward as you stretch your arm. Make sure that you do not stretch out your arm too much—the elbow should still be soft rather than locked.

4

When you have extended your arm as far as feels comfortable, inhale and slowly lift your left arm again, moving it back in a semi-circular motion the other way until it is resting by your side with your palm flat on the floor. At the same time, bring your right leg back up to its starting position, with the knee bent and the foot flat on the floor.

Tip

Keep your head centered and do not let it drop to the side during this exercise. Keep looking up at the ceiling as you move.

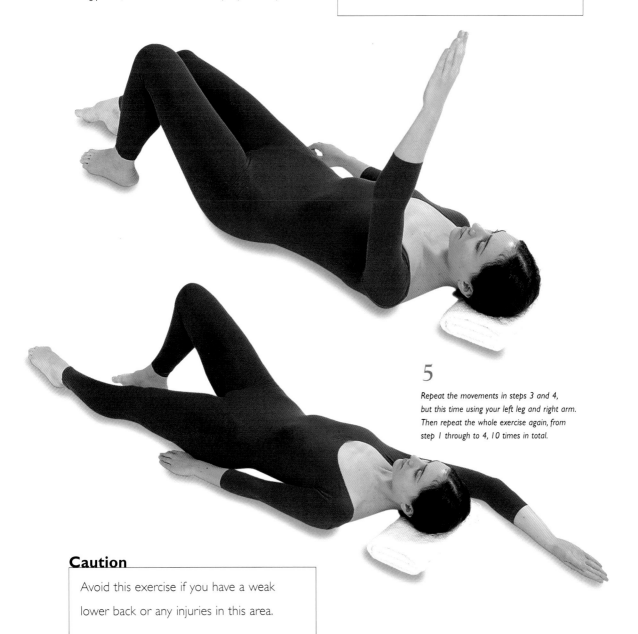

5

Repeat the movements in steps 3 and 4, but this time using your left leg and right arm. Then repeat the whole exercise again, from step 1 through to 4, 10 times in total.

Caution

Avoid this exercise if you have a weak lower back or any injuries in this area.

Hip and thigh toner

This excellent exercise helps to stretch and tone the quadriceps, or thigh muscles. It will improve flexibility and increase strength at the front of your hip and the knee. You will need a small pillow, cushion, or folded towel.

1

Lie on the floor on your left side, and extend your left arm out on the floor behind your head with your left palm flat on the floor. Place the pillow or towel on the upper part of your left arm, and then rest the left side of your head on it. Allow your right arm to rest in front of your body in line with your shoulder, with the palm flat on the floor. Bend your knees to an angle of about 45 degrees.

2

Pull in your navel toward your spine and pull up your pelvic floor. Hold them in that position, then release them slightly and hold them at about 25 per cent of the tension. Keep breathing rhythmically, using the thoracic breathing method (see page 23).

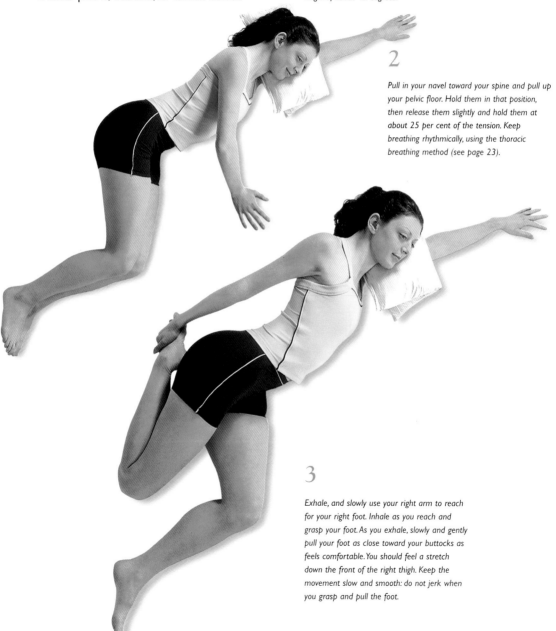

3

Exhale, and slowly use your right arm to reach for your right foot. Inhale as you reach and grasp your foot. As you exhale, slowly and gently pull your foot as close toward your buttocks as feels comfortable. You should feel a stretch down the front of the right thigh. Keep the movement slow and smooth: do not jerk when you grasp and pull the foot.

Caution

If you feel any pain in your hip, thigh or knee during this exercise, stop at once and seek qualified medical advice.

4

Now inhale and gently release the stretch on the leg, moving the leg back toward its original position. Repeat this stretch 10 times in total, exhaling on each stretch.

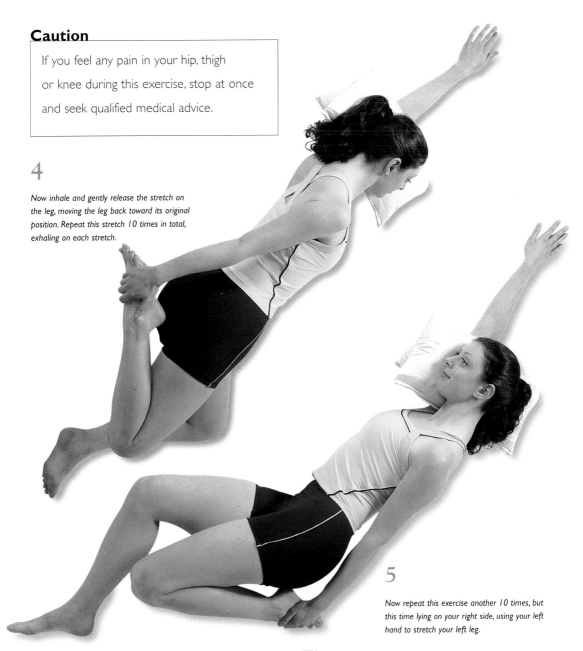

5

Now repeat this exercise another 10 times, but this time lying on your right side, using your left hand to stretch your left leg.

Tip

Keep your abdominal muscles pulled in throughout. Do not let your back arch or your head turn away from the pillow.

GLOSSARY

Adrenaline
A hormone secreted by the adrenal gland, which prepares the body for "fight or flight." It has widespread effects on the muscles, circulation and sugar metabolism.

Alignment
Positioned in a straight line.

Biceps
This term is most often used for the muscles at the front of the upper arms, but there are also biceps at the back of the thighs.

Carbon dioxide
A colourless gas formed in the tissues during metabolism, which is carried in the blood to the lungs and then exhaled.

Centering
This term refers to the technique of centering the body by strengthening and stabilizing the powerhouse (the area from the abdominal muscles to the buttocks, which stretches round the body at the back and the front).

Cervical lordosis
A postural problem of the spine that occurs in the neck area. The muscles at the back of the neck contract, while those at the front overexpand. The chin protrudes forward and over time this condition can cause inflammation of the joints, including arthritis.

Ch'i
According to Chinese tradition, this energy, or "life force," permeates everything—it is within and around all things, living or otherwise.

Cortisol
This is a steroid hormone produced in the body that is important for normal stress-response and carbohydrate metabolism.

Deltoids
These are the thick triangular muscles that cover the shoulder joints—they are responsible for raising up the arms from the sides of the body.

Ectomorph
One of three basic body shapes—the other two are endomorph and mesomorph. Ectomorph people tend to be light and delicate, often tall and thin with long limbs. This body shape is often linked to an alert, inhibited and intellectual personality.

Endomorph
One of the three basic body shapes. People with this body shape will be heavy or rounded, and may have trouble keeping their body weight down. This shape is quite often linked to placidity, a relaxed attitude and hedonism.

Endorphins
"Happy" chemicals that occur naturally in the brain and have pain-relieving qualities. They are also responsible for feelings of pleasure.

Fight-or-flight response
A process that prepares the body for physical effort. When the body is under extreme stress, it gears up to meet the immediate threat by releasing adrenaline and other hormones into the system. The heartbeat, metabolism and breathing become more rapid, and any bodily function that is not essential to immediate survival—including the immune system and digestion processes—are automatically shut down.

Gluteus maximus
These paired muscles are located within the fleshy part of the buttocks.

Gluteus minimus
These are the paired muscles situated above the fleshy part of the buttocks.

Levator scapulis
Muscles at the sides and back of the neck.

Leucocytes
White blood cells that help to protect the body against foreign substances and disease.

Lumbar lordosis
A postural problem of the spine in which the abdominal muscles are weakened, pulling the stomach forward and creating an unnatural inward curve in the lower back.

Lymph
The name for the fluid present in the lymphatic system (a network of vessels). Lymph carries leucocytes, or white blood cells, which play a key role in helping the body to fight off disease.

Mesomorph
One of the three basic body shapes. People with this body shape will be athletic or muscular, with large chests, limbs and muscles. This body shape is sometimes associated with an aggressive tendency. Mesomorphs are often athletic and excel at sports.

Powerhouse
The area from the abdominal muscles to our buttocks, stretching round the body. In Pilates, this is the area from which all energy and effort travel outward.

Quadriceps
Muscles situated in the thighs.

Rickets
A disease of childhood in which the bones do not harden and become soft and malformed. It is caused by a deficiency of vitamin D.

Swayback
A postural problem where the thoracic spine becomes distorted and results in weak ligaments and muscles.

T'ai Chi Ch'uan
This is a flowing form of movement, working on mind, body and spirit, which dates back to China at least 2,000 years.

T'an Tien
The Chinese word for the reservoir of ch'i energy situated in the abdominal area.

Thoracic breathing
Sometimes known as "lateral breathing." This technique involves breathing into the back and lower ribs: as the air goes into the lungs, the back and sides of the rib cage expand, then they contract as the air is exhaled. In this way, the abdomen can stay contracted and tight and yet not interfere with the intake of breath.

Thoracic kyphosis
This is a postural problem that causes excessive outward curvature of the spine and eventual hunching of the back.

Thoracic straight spine
This is a postural problem that causes the spine to straighten as a result of muscle contraction. It causes pain in the arms and strain in the chest area.

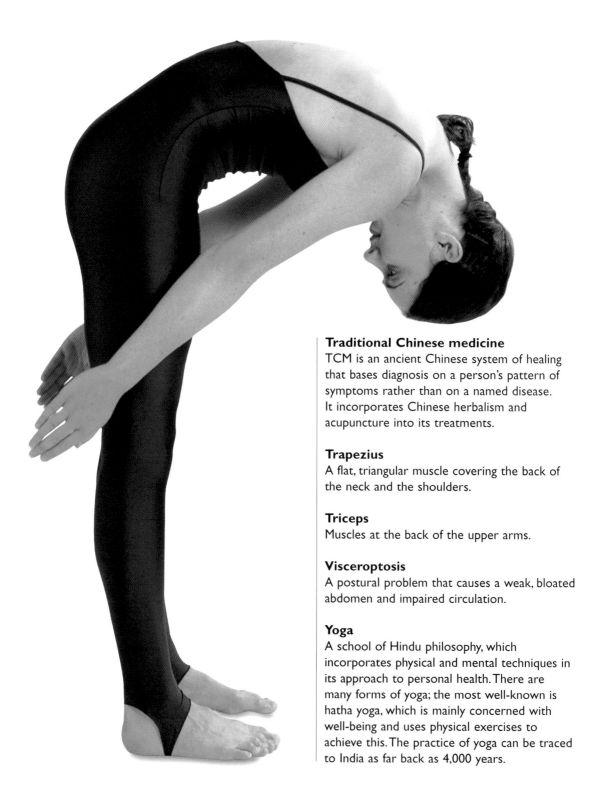

Traditional Chinese medicine
TCM is an ancient Chinese system of healing that bases diagnosis on a person's pattern of symptoms rather than on a named disease. It incorporates Chinese herbalism and acupuncture into its treatments.

Trapezius
A flat, triangular muscle covering the back of the neck and the shoulders.

Triceps
Muscles at the back of the upper arms.

Visceroptosis
A postural problem that causes a weak, bloated abdomen and impaired circulation.

Yoga
A school of Hindu philosophy, which incorporates physical and mental techniques in its approach to personal health. There are many forms of yoga; the most well-known is hatha yoga, which is mainly concerned with well-being and uses physical exercises to achieve this. The practice of yoga can be traced to India as far back as 4,000 years.

Useful addresses and websites

The Pilates Center

4800 Baseline Road, Suite D206

Boulder, CO 80303

Telephone: 303 494 3400

Fax: 303 494 5151

info@thepilatescenter.com

The Pilates Center of Austin

5555 N. Lamar Boulevard, Suite E103

Austin, Texas 78751

Telephone: 512 467 8009

info@pilatescenterofaustin.com

Alternative Health & Fitness Concepts

2016 Walnut Street, 2nd floor

Philadelphia, PA 19103

1-877-9 Pilates

Telephone: 215 567 4969

Fax: 215 567 4881

Pilates Method Alliance

2631 Lincoln Avenue

Miami, FL 33133

Telephone: 866 573 4945

www.pilatesmethodalliance.org

Body Balance

1009 North Rush Street, 4th floor

Chicago, IL 60611

Telephone: 312 440 9558

www.bodybalanceltd.com

Every Body Pilates

454 Common St.

Belmont, MA 02478

Telephone: 617 484 3311

www.everybodypilates.com

Index

abdominal muscles 26, 37, 59
adrenal gland 60
adrenaline 12, 21, 60
aerobics 11
alignment 60
arched back 59

backward swimming 56
balance 8, 10
biceps 14, 60
body shapes 7
bones 15
breathing
    abdominal 23
    correct 22
    shallow 23

carbon dioxide 60
centering 26, 60
cervical lordosis 29, 60
cervical vertebrae 15
ch'i 26, 60
chest stretches see exercises
circulation 10
clavicle 15
clothing 17
coccyx 15
cortisol 60

deltoids 14, 60
digestion 10

ectomorph 7, 60
emotions 12
endomorph 7, 60
endorphins 21, 60
equipment 16, 24, 44, 56
exercises
    arm swings 34–35
    backward swimming 56
    chest stretch 44, 54
    head lift 33
    hip and thigh toner 58
    knee bends and arm lifts 42
    large hoops 36
    lumbar twists 52
    progressive hoops 37
    sitting 46–49
    small hoops 36
    spinal release 45
    spinal twists 48

standing exercises 38–45
    warming up 34
expectant mothers 18

fat-burning exercise 20
femur 15
fibula 15
fight or flight response 12, 21, 60

gluteus maximus 14, 60
gluteus minimus 14, 61

head lift see exercises 33
high blood pressure 45
hip and thigh toner see exercises
humerus 15

immune system 10

knee bends and arm lifts see exercises
kung fu 26

large hoops see exercises
lateral breathing see thoracic breathing
leucocytes 61
levator scapulis 14, 61
lower back 46, 48, 57
    pain 51
lumbar lordosis 29, 62
lumbar twists see exercises
lumbar vetebrae 15
lymph 62

mandible 15
matwork 50–59
mesomorph 7, 61
metabolism 60
metacarpals 15
metatarsals 15
muscles 14

nerves 13
neutral position 51, 54

patella 15
pelvic floor muscle 39, 42, 44, 45, 46, 51, 52, 54, 58
phalanges 15
Pilates, history and development 8–9
Pilates, Joseph 6, 8
postural habits 28

posture 28, 29, 30, 38
    bad 29, 30
    correct 38, 50
    standing correctly 38
"powerhouse" of the body 26, 27, 46, 61
progressive hoops see exercises

quadriceps 14, 61

radius 15
ribs 15
rickets 61

sacrum 15
safety 18
scapula 15
shoulder blades 46
sitting correctly 46
sitting exercises see exercises
skull 15
small hoops see exercises
spinal problems 29
spinal release see exercises
spinal twists see exercises
spine 42
sports mat 16
standing correctly 38
standing exercises see exercises
sternum 15
swayback 29, 61

t'ai chi ch'uan 4, 26, 61
t'an tien 26, 61
tarsals 15
thoracic breathing 23, 24, 27, 36, 39, 42, 45, 47, 48, 51, 52, 54, 56, 58, 61
thoracic kyphosis 29, 61
thoracic straight spine 29, 61
thoracic vertebrae 15
tibia 15
tissue (body) 13
traditional Chinese medicine 62
trapezius 14, 62
triceps 14, 62

ulna 15

visualization 21

yoga 6, 62